End

In reading this book, you will experience God's faithfulness in leading this family through years in the wilderness of terror, despair, and anger with God. The result: four faith warriors who are able to truly say, "God is good!"

—Dr. Barbara Oats
Ph.D., NCC, LPCC

This book reminds us that even today ordinary people can rely on an extraordinary God and amazing things happen.

—Jerilyn Renner

Mike and Laura Roberts and their sons, Cole and Clay, have experienced life's deep waters of difficulty and suffering. Many who find themselves in challenging circumstances often give up, but this is the story of a family that didn't give up! The Roberts family is a modern-day example of those who choose to fight the good fight of faith and not give up.

Laura has a beautiful way of communicating how God strengthened their family through an incredibly challenging journey . . . You will be amazed at the miracles they experienced at just the right time, and the scriptures that became an anchor in their tough times will certainly inspire you.

—Pastor Doug and Vicki Graham

By Faith

By Faith

A Family's Search For Meaning In Suffering

Laura Roberts

TATE PUBLISHING & *Enterprises*

Published by Tate Publishing & Enterprises, LLC
127 E. Trade Center Terrace | Mustang, Oklahoma 73064 USA
1.888.361.9473 | www.tatepublishing.com

Tate Publishing is committed to excellence in the publishing industry. The company reflects the philosophy established by the founders, based on Psalm 68:11,
"The Lord gave the word and great was the company of those who published it."

Book design copyright © 2009 by Tate Publishing, LLC. All rights reserved.
Cover design by Amber Lee
Interior design by Jeff Fisher

Published in the United States of America

ISBN: 978-1-60799-836-5
1. Biography, Autobiography, Personal Memoirs
2. Health & Fitness, Childrens Health
09.07.21

Dedication

To Mike, the love of my life. Thank you for being a wonderful husband and father. I am so glad that God has chosen you to be my life partner. You are my rock that helps hold me up through all we have been through. I am so very grateful for the support you have given to me during the writing of this book. It has been hard to relive some of the painful times, but I have made it through with your unending love. I cannot wait to see the next journey that God has in store for us, and I know with you alongside me, both doing God's will, all will be fine.

To Cole and Clay, my wonderful boys, thank you for being so brave by allowing me to write about the good, bad, painful, and joyful times in your lives. I am so proud of you for allowing the stories to be told so God may be honored and get the glory for our lives that he deserves. Also, I hope others will find peace on their journey, which will lead them to a strong relationship with God. I love you both so very much, and I am proud to be the mother of such amazing young men who have a heart for and a deep desire to serve the Lord. May God bless you both in all you do in this life.

Through the writing of this book, I have come to recognize the suffering all three of you have endured. I am so sorry it has taken this long and the writing of this book to really allow it to sink in. I pray this book will be as healing for you as it has been for me. I love you!

Acknowledgments

To Lisa Leingang, without your willingness to use the great gift of writing that God has given you, this book would not have been possible. Thank you so very much for all the time you put into this book with me, not only as my friend who kept encouraging me, but also as the one who would take the words I had written down and help make them be honorable to God. I truly believe God brought us together to share this story for his glory.

May God bless you and your family for all your work and obedience to his calling. I pray that all the wonderful stories you have written that speak of and show God's gracious hand in our lives be one day published for all to read and truly enjoy. God has given you a blessed gift of showing himself to others through your writing, and I am deeply grateful and honored to have you be a part of this book becoming a reality.

Special Thank You

To my Father in heaven, nothing would have been possible without your loving hand. It is through your wonderful guidance and love for us that all has been accomplished.

To my family and friends, without all of you, we as a family could not have made it through all that we have. You are all truly a blessing!

To all who have touched our lives, thank you for being a part of our journey in all the big and small ways. Every one of you has made such a difference.

To Lisa, thank you again for all you and your family have done to help make this book become a reality.

To Doreen Schumacher, thank you for allowing me to share the blessed story of the heartbreaking death of your son, all in hopes to bring glory to God and comfort to others.

Table of Contents

Foreword

Take a walk with Laura Roberts. The path she leads you on is filled with fearful anxiety and devastation. Keep walking and you will notice that with every heartbreaking calamity there is an astonishing victory. Soon you will see that she does not walk alone.

Directly from the heart of a mother, this fascinating true story of one family and their battles with blindness, cancer, heart surgery, and more is told with brutal honesty as Laura finds herself wondering... *where is God?*

On this same path, God reveals himself through incredible miracles that go hand-in-hand with every tragedy. His presence becomes clearer with every step that is taken down this troubled road, and Laura is given strength in the knowledge that *God is here.*

In a world that believes the miracles of biblical times no longer exist, this book is a shining reminder that God is present and still in control. Laura's story needs to be heard not only by those who are struggling with difficulties but also by those who are struggling to know that God is in fact still with us.

—Lisa Leingang

Introduction

This is a true story of my family's life that I told with my heart and my perception of what happened. I will be introducing you to my husband, Mike, a wonderful husband, father, and best friend; Cole, who is blind and a cancer survivor, and who has also undergone over fifty-two surgeries in his thirteen years of life, with many miracles from God; and Clay, my youngest, who has shown his great courage and love for God through heart surgery, allergies, and asthma.

When I started to journal, I was pregnant with Cole. I never dreamed I would be able to take that journal and make it into a book. Who would have thought that my life and my family's life would have been so filled with hardship and miracles that a book could be made?

As I sat thinking about what I would like you to know, some thoughts came into my mind: *Did I want this life? Is this my childhood dream and fantasy of what my family would be like?* The answer to this would first have to be an honest no! But believe me, as fast as that no would leave my lips, the yes would already be emerging. Please know I would not want the pain and suffering my children have endured; I would change that. But to think of my life without them, I cannot.

I am grateful for all that happened, as I feel it has all blessed us in so many ways already, and I know deep down there will be many more blessings to come. I think to myself: *Without this journey, would we be as close to each other as we are? Would God be as big a part in our lives as he is? Would we be the people we are now, growing daily from our mistakes and repenting for them?* I can honestly say, I do not know! I want to say *yes* to these questions, but deep in my heart I am who I am today because of my journey and allowing God to be my guide in this life, not my humanness.

I know God had his hand on us from the beginning and before this journey started. He has kept us going when we humanly should not have been able to. I have learned that I must start my faith in him anew every day; I cannot live on yesterday's faith alone.

I am writing this story to bring glory to God. You will *witness* his wonderful miracles in our daily lives as a family who struggles with many difficult situations. This book not only tells our story, but it is a testimony to the fact that no matter what life gives you, all things are possible with the help of God. I want you to see how strong our boys are physically, emotionally, and spiritually so that you may know that no matter how small you are, God is with you and will help you through all things if you truly surrender yourself to him. My hope is that this book will be an encouraging resource to assist you along your personal journey. May it bring you great comfort to know that you are not alone on your walk.

The Birth of Cole

All through history, mothers have felt grief, anxiety, and worry, all because of this powerful instinct called "a mother's love." From the time Abel died at the hands of his brother, mothers have had struggles and trials resulting from the love they hold for their children. Imagine Sarah's grief as she watched her husband, Abraham, lead their only long-awaited son up the mountain, knowing he was to be the sacrifice (Gen 22). It would be days before she would find out that God spared her boy. Now imagine the heartbreak of Moses' mother as she watched her baby float away from her down the river (Ex 2). Her only hope was her faith that God would be his protector.

I am one of these mothers. Although my story may be different from theirs, it is the same. We share the same terrifying moments of the unknown and the same triumphant joy in personal victories.

When my husband, Mike, and I decided it was time to start a family, I was ecstatic at the very thought of having a baby. When I became pregnant, we were thrilled. Our minds were filled with wonderful thoughts of this baby and the family it would be starting. Sadly, that pregnancy ended in a miscarriage. The heartbreak of losing our first child was followed by two painful years of being unable to conceive again. We tried everything possible to make another pregnancy happen. Tests, consultations, more tests; it was physically draining and the waiting was frustrating.

So many couples around us were having children, some who didn't even plan for them, yet we had been waiting so long and still nothing. I knew in my heart I would be a good mom, and Mike would be a wonderful father. We both had so much love to give, so why not us? It was a strain on our emotions and on our marriage. But then, it happened! Our first miracle of many to come. I became pregnant, and both the baby and I were healthy. I felt God's blessing inside of me and rejoiced in it.

Of the many happy days of pregnancy, there was one that sticks out in my memory. I was walking with a friend of mine at the mall. Actually, I was waddling more than walking because I was in my last trimester and was fairly big. We went past a group of severely handicapped children. I watched them briefly in their wheelchairs, unable to move other than the jerks and twitches their bodies performed on their own. My heart went out to them as I consciously rubbed my large, protruding belly.

"I could not deal with that," I confided to the friend I was walking with. Funny how limited we see ourselves. If only I knew what God had planned for me and this baby I was so tenderly caressing. If only I realized what God was calling me to deal with and the amazing blessings that would be produced.

I was working nights in a beauty salon so that when the baby was born either Mike or I would be home to take care of him. It was important to us that our child would not need to go to a day care or have a full-time babysitter. We simply wanted him to be surrounded by those who loved him the most at all times of his life.

I had just finished a nine-hour shift on my feet,

cutting and styling hair for my clients. I came home tired, so I took a calm, relaxing bath while Mike was on the phone talking to his sister, Laura (Yes, his sister is a Laura too!), about a trip to France that she was getting ready for. "What would you like me to bring back for you from France?" Laura had asked Mike.

"I don't know," answered Mike. "What do you think?"

"I was thinking maybe some holy water," she answered.

I was not aware of their conversation because my attention was focused on the fact that my water had just broken. "Water!" I yelled from the bathroom.

Mike heard me yell and answered his sister. "Yes, Laura agrees. You should bring back some holy water."

"Water!" I yelled again, wondering why Mike had not dropped the phone and come running.

"Yes, I heard you," he hollered back to me. "I told her to bring water."

Confused and frustrated at that point, I yelled again, "Water! My water broke!"

"Her water broke!" Mike yelled into the phone.

"Her water broke?" my sister-in-law answered. "That's a sign! Holy water it is!"

At 5:33 p.m. on January 13, 1995, Cole Estes Roberts was born. At that moment, I praised and thanked God for such a miracle. When I looked down at that little baby in my arms, I knew I was looking at an angel.

She conceived again, and when she gave birth to a son, she said, "This time I will praise the Lord."

Genesis 29:35

The Search for Answers

The first time I felt a twinge that something might be wrong was when the doctor commented on the umbilical cord as he was examining it. "That's funny," he said. "There are only two blood vessels, and there should be three. I guess I will find out more after the lab checks it." For a split second I felt fear, and my stomach did a flip. That fear melted away, however, as soon as I held the baby we had waited so long for.

I was in the tub the next day when the nurse came in and said Cole could not be circumcised because he had hypospadias. (This is a birth defect where the opening of the urethra is on the underside of the penis instead of at the tip.) She said, "A lot of boys have this. Don't worry." When she left, I began to cry. Despite the nurse's reassuring words, I felt something was seriously wrong; however, because it was just a feeling that only I was aware of, I felt horribly scared and alone.

The doctor later explained that hypospadias was a fairly common occurrence; about three in every one thousand boys have this condition. Cole would have to have surgery to fix this problem when he was a little older. I was nervous and worried, as any first-time mom would be, while the doctor discussed the concerns and conditions involving this sweet new life. I prayed passionately that when it was time for surgery all would go well and my newborn would not experience any pain. Ironically, Cole's first surgery was not to fix the hypospadias. I was changing his diaper and found a lump in his groin area. It turned out to be a hernia. When he was only six weeks old, he had to have surgery to fix it.

It was the first time I had to let my baby go and trust him in the hands of strangers. I could not see, let alone control, what was happening on the other side of those swinging doors. He was so little and helpless, and he needed his mother. Even though that thought haunted me, I was thinking even more about whether I would be able to perform his aftercare in the best way possible. I wasn't a nurse; I was still trying to figure out how to take care of a baby, let alone a baby who just had surgery.

When the surgery was over and I was able to take him home, I was terrified. I did not want to leave the help of the nurses, but Mike was with me and we would work as a team. Mike was terrified that he might hurt Cole, so it was up to me to figure out Cole's aftercare. Don't get me wrong, I was scared stiff too, but diapers needed changing.

The next few weeks were a mass of emotional confusion for me. Cole cried whenever I would lay him down and sometimes even when we would just touch him too quickly. Needless to say, he never seemed to sleep. I couldn't shake the feeling that something was wrong, so I took him to several doctors several times. They all just told me he was a colicky baby. Well, yes, I have heard of babies with colic and how they are fussy and don't sleep, but I thought to myself, *Come on, this cannot be what they are talking about.* I was a brand new mom, so what did I really know? Certainly the doctors with their years of experience and education would know best. At least, that is what I kept telling myself; however, Cole continued to cry constantly. I could not help but feel like a complete failure. Why did I not know how to make Cole feel better? I was his mother; where were those maternal instincts that should show me how to comfort my own child? I continually asked God to give me those motherly instincts. I became so frustrated when I could not calm Cole down. I kept thinking God was not answering my prayers.

What I did not know then was that he had indeed answered my payers even before I had prayed them. It was the motherly instincts he had given me that kept telling me something was seriously wrong, but I forced myself to believe in the doctors' answers instead of what I felt to be true.

Be strong, and let your heart take courage, all you who hope in the Lord.

Psalm 31:24 NLT

"I have much more to say to you, more than you can now bear. But when he, the Spirit of truth, comes, he will guide you into all truth. He will not speak on his own; he will speak only what he hears, and he will tell you what is yet to come."

John 16:12–13

A Point of Desperation

Things were getting worse as the weeks went on. Cole was throwing up a lot and never seemed to want to open his eyes. I took him to more doctors, and every one of them still labeled me as being an overly worried new mom.

My frustration increased to the point of desperation. My boss had told me about a neonatal doctor that she knew of. I didn't even make an appointment; I just rushed to his office. I felt like I was in a fog as I walked into the hospital where he worked. I practically begged for him to look at my baby. Praise God, this wonderful man agreed to see my Cole.

My heart raced as I watched how he examined Cole. He spent a lot of time observing his eyes. He turned the lights on and off. He touched Cole's arms and legs to see what his reaction would be. What did all this mean? It was obvious he spotted something that concerned him ... but what? While he was still looking into Cole's eyes, he told me to call my husband and have him come to the hospital. What could all this be? What was wrong with my baby?

I felt sick to my stomach and my hands shook as I dialed Mike's number. After what seemed like an eternity, Mike walked through the doorway. I could see the worry on his face as well. When we were both there, the doctor explained that he was not quite sure what was wrong but felt it was possible that Cole might have a brain tumor (neuroblastoma) or possibly another very rare condition. The doctor would need to do more research before he could talk to us about what that other possibility might be.

My heart sank to my feet, and I felt like throwing up. We could not believe what he was telling us. Questions began swirling in my mind: *Could I have caused this? What could I have done differently?* Despair, anger, terror, and a thousand other emotions clawed at me. Feeling such helplessness, what could and would I do? *Pray!* I prayed while the doctor continued to talk about options. I prayed while we walked to where they had Cole. I didn't even know what to pray; I just knew I needed to connect with God. By the time I found myself in the chapel of that hospital, I knew what I wanted to communicate to God about through my prayers. *Please, please, God, heal my baby; make this all go away!*

The days were long and filled with many tests on Cole. I did not sleep at all, for my place was with my baby. The results of all the testing were bittersweet. Cole did not have neuroblastoma on the brain; *thank you, God!* What Cole was diagnosed with was a condition called aniridia/wilms.

Aniridia is a rare condition one is born with. This condition is characterized by the lack of an iris in the eye. Aniridia literally means without iris. It never occurred to us that Cole did not have an iris. We simply thought he had very dark eyes. Aniridia is just one symptom of a genetic disorder called WAGR. To be diagnosed with WAGR, the patient must have at least two of these four symptoms:

W—Wilms tumor: malignant cancer of the kidneys

A—Aniridia: no iris

<u>G</u>—Genital and/or urinary tract abnormalities

<u>R</u>—Mental retardation/developmental disabilities

Cole at this point only had two symptoms—aniridia and genital abnormalities. In my heart I thought that was too much.

Because aniridia dealt with the eyes, it was only logical that Cole would be seen by an eye doctor; however, I was not prepared for the doctor that would be checking out our precious little boy. His bedside manner was appalling. He had to examine Cole by placing some metal clips into his eyes to hold them open, and he was not gentle about it at all. He had no soothing words or gentle touch for Cole. He simply did his job.

We were not allowed to be with Cole in the doctor's room. All we could do was pace back and forth together outside the door listening to him scream for thirty minutes straight. Looking for a glimpse of reassurance that we were doing the right thing by letting this doctor examine Cole, Mike and I looked through the neonatal window at Mike's parents and my dad, who were waiting nervously in the hallway. Unfortunately, this did not bring us any peace. If only at this time I could have put my trust and peace in God. When we were finally able to go in, Cole looked like he just had a bath. His clothes were soaked with sweat and bloody tears from crying so hard. At last Cole simply fell asleep from pure exhaustion.

When all was finished, this horrid doctor stood in front of Mike and me and quite matter-of-factly said, "He is blind; you should take him home." Then he walked out the door. The neonatal doctor immediately apologized for the actions of the eye doctor, and as he continued to tell us to not worry, his words became like background noise to me. At that very moment, everything just stopped. It felt as though I had left my body and was watching it all from above. I could not breathe. I had to get out, get away. I ran so fast, not even knowing where I was going. I was oblivious to everyone around me, including my father, who was calling after me. I did not notice Mike falling into the arms of his parents, who had to hold him up. Mike and I could not comfort each other because we could not control our own actions.

I found myself once again in the chapel, where I flung myself onto the floor, barely able to hear my own screams. I tried to quiet those screams and sobs, but it was too painful to hold them down. My heart was gone, ripped from me, so why did I feel every beat as if it would explode? I had to concentrate on not throwing up. I had to concentrate on not acting crazy. I felt as though my baby's life got torn away before he even had a chance to live. I equated the diagnoses of the loss of his sight with the loss of his very life.

This all happened in minutes, but it seemed like hours before my dad found me. He scooped me up and held me like he did when I was a child. I wanted to pray, but I just could not. Instead, I yelled at God to heal my son. I shouted out, "Why? Oh, God, why?" over and over as my father rocked me and gently stroked my hair saying, "It will be okay; it will be okay."

In my distress I called to the Lord; I called out to my God. From his temple he heard my voice; my cry came to his ears.

2 Samuel 22:7

Major Surgery for Baby Cole

My world suddenly became a search for knowledge. We needed to know exactly what Cole's condition was and what we required to deal with it. We needed to know how to take care of our son. The doctors who specialized in Cole's conditions were located in Arizona and Minnesota. We decided to go to the doctors in Arizona because my parents lived there and we would have a place to stay.

The testing began immediately. For one test in particular, they had wrapped Cole's little legs in cellophane so tightly that they had turned purple. From the intensity of Cole's cries, I knew he had to be in a lot of pain. I could not stand to see him that way. I had to leave the room. My dad was with us at that appointment, and he could not take it much longer either. He picked Cole up to comfort him and demanded that the wrappings be taken off immediately.

When I left the room, I walked aimlessly though the halls of the hospital and saw a lot of disabled and very sick children. This triggered thoughts of what I might have to deal with as Cole got older. I felt I needed some questions answered, so I called a friend of mine who was in nursing school at the time. I do not remember the questions I had for her, but I do remember her words to me. She told me that Cole might be hanging on to life just for me. She told me I should be a little less selfish and tell him it is okay for him to go home.

I thought about what she said and walked back to his room with the intention of doing what she had suggested. Cole and I were alone when I looked down at my precious baby lying in his crib. I wanted to tell him it was okay to let go. I wanted to tell him he could go home, but I could not. The more I pondered what I had been told, the more I thought my friend had it backwards. I felt it would be selfish of me to let him go just because I thought I could not deal with a disabled child. Who was I to play God or even think I had that kind of power to tell Cole when to go home? As I continued to think, I could not imagine telling him it was okay to die because I could not, nor did I want to, live my life without him. I never told anyone about that conversation I had with my friend. I was embarrassed about even thinking of asking Cole to let go and go home.

The doctors were looking for the cancerous growth neuroblastoma throughout the entirety of Cole's body. To do this, they had to give Cole one shot of radiation every day for three days straight. On that third day, I picked up my baby and was horrified to see all of his beautiful dark hair still lying on his little pillow. At that moment, I was hit hard with the realization of just how serious this could be, and I couldn't help but wonder how long my child would be with us in this world. After what seemed like forever, we finally were able to leave the hospital, and the sad thing was, I knew nothing more than when I got there except I now had the horrifying pictures that will be forever ingrained in my mind of all the painful testing Cole had to endure.

As soon as we got back to my parents' house, I took Cole to the eye doctor for his first examination. She confirmed what we had already been told—that Cole had aniridia.

One of the symptoms of aniridia is that all the tube-like parts in the body are smaller than normal. This makes drainage the body does naturally difficult, and pressure can build up. In the human eye, the iris meets with the white part of the eye, which is called the drainage angle. This is where the fluid of the inner eye drains. (Not to be confused with tear ducts. Tears lubricate the outer surface of the eye.)

After the examination, the doctor told us Cole would need to have surgery right away, as the pressure in his left eye was very high. As she explained what she would be doing, my heart ached and my stomach flipped. All I kept thinking about was her operating on his tiny eye.

On the way back to my parents' house, I tried to put all the fear I was feeling aside so Cole would not pick up on my emotions. That night I lay in bed and so many thoughts raced in and out of my mind uncontrollably as I cried—would the doctor make a mistake and Cole would end up blind, did I make the right doctor choice, or should I get a second opinion, to please, God, please, heal him tonight as he sleeps.

On April 3, 1995, I handed Cole over to the doctor for the first of many eye surgeries. I will never forget the feeling of complete loss when they took him from me, and no matter how hard I tried, I could not stop the endless flow of tears. Even though the doctor talked to me before surgery and explained what she was going to do, I felt no peace. The doctors would put a flap on the drainage angle of the eye to allow the inner eye fluid to drain and relieve the pressure that was building up in his eye.

During surgery I remember praying what I can describe to you as a chant, as I just kept saying over and over, "God, please heal him and guide the doctors." Some of the prayers even became a bargaining act: "God, if you heal him I promise to do this and never do that." As I write this down, I realize how young I was in my faith walk with God. If I only could have had the ability to surrender all my fears and trust in his plan as I do today. Then I realize that this immense journey and all its insecurities has made me who I am today in Christ.

After surgery Cole had to wear a patch over the eye that was worked on, and I was really impressed that he didn't keep trying to take it off. As for me, I did not want the patch to come off because I was too scared to see what was underneath it, and as long as it was on, I felt the eye was protected.

Nine days later, on April 12, 1995, Cole had glaucoma surgery again. Mike was not able to be with us while that surgery took place. He had to stay home in North Dakota to work. This was really hard for him, as his baby boy was going through the trauma of an operation and he was unable to give the love and comfort he so much wanted to give. Not having Mike there to face this with me and having to endure the waiting room without the strong hand of my best friend was very difficult for me; however, I felt very much in control with what was going on medically. I was trying to stay on top of it all so I could make the best choices possible for Cole.

Looking back at this time, I came to the realization that I was a great hider. I had nothing in control.

I remember sitting on the couch once we got back to my parents' house from surgery and just holding Cole and crying, praying, "Please, God, give us a miracle; help us because I do not want to do this anymore."

After Cole's glaucoma surgery, we were able to finally come home. Mike and I were thrilled to be together as a family again, but the thrill did not last long. As soon as we got home, Cole had to be hospitalized for influenza. Although we were all in the same town once more, we were unable to enjoy each other in our home. I stayed at the hospital with Cole night and day. Mike would come to be with Cole when he was not working, and I would take that opportunity to go home and shower.

When Cole was released from the hospital, we did have a couple of weeks to be together at home as a family. It was so nice to finally put Cole to sleep in his own room that we worked so hard to get ready for him. I remember just sitting in the room looking at the crib Mike put together and the brightly colored clowns that we had painted on the wall. Nothing felt so peaceful in such a long time than that very moment. Then as soon as it came it went.

It was time to say good-bye to Daddy once again and fly back to Arizona. Cole had an ultrasound done on his kidneys to make sure there were no Wilms cancer tumors. This cancer can be a symptom of WAGR, so Cole would have to have these ultrasounds done every three months. One positive outlook was that Cole did not mind the ultrasounds and there was no pain involved with them at all. This was one of the first times I felt okay with a test that Cole would have to endure frequently in his life. I felt God's presence and voice telling me, "I am here and will never leave you."

On June 16, 1995, Cole had tubes put into his ears because he was getting a lot of ear infections. This again is a result of the small drainage tubes in children with aniridia.

Another common trait of children with aniridia is throwing up on a regular basis. To prevent this, Cole had major surgery, called a fundoplication, done on June 21, 1995; he was only six months old. It was strange to me that this surgery would have the title of *major* in front of it. Every surgery performed on this little baby was major. But if by *major* it was meant that it would be longer, more painful, and more emotionally traumatic, then I would say this title was an understatement.

The intention of that surgery was to tie Cole's stomach around his esophagus so that it would be impossible for him to throw up.

The night before the surgery was very difficult. Cole had a tube put down his nose and into his throat to measure acid backup. The tube itself naturally bothered Cole, and to make things worse, he was hungry because he could not eat or drink for twelve hours. As I watched Mike hold him and Cole being so uncomfortable, I just started to pray with everything I had inside of me. "Please, God, let him fall asleep; let him feel comfort." God is so good because Cole, even though still miserable, was able to rest for short periods of time. Looking at his little face with his eyes closed resting on his dad's shoulder was such a great gift from God. As for the surgery itself, Cole had to be opened up from mid-chest to his belly button for the doctors to work on him.

After the surgery, he was in intensive care for a week. I thank God that this surgery was done in town so Mike could be with us the whole time. I am not sure how I would have held up alone. Cole was in so much pain we could not even hold him. There were tubes everywhere, and all Mike and I could do for him was take turns holding his hand and just touching him so he would know we were there. All the doctors could do at that point was keep him comfortable. The minute Cole would start to cry, they would give him more pain medication.

I have often heard of people wanting to change places with a hurting loved one, and it was then that I truly understood that view. I felt horrible that my baby had to go through so much and I had no way of changing it. I just wanted to scoop him up; the desire of a mother wanting desperately to hold her baby and make the hurt go away was so strong. I was disturbed by the fact that I had allowed it in the first place. I prayed Cole would never remember this pain. I would watch him lying there, helpless, and there I was by his side, helpless. Knowing my arms around him would hurt him, I asked God to send his son, Jesus, to hold our son, Cole, so that he would feel his peace and not the pain.

It felt so good to be able to hold him again when we were able to do so. We were very nervous about taking him home. He had a lot of stitches, so we had to be careful; and again, I was worried about my responsibilities with his aftercare. I had no choice, and I knew in my heart that God would help me know what I needed to do. When we got home, I did my best to be as gentle as I could when tending to his stitches and taking care of him. He was so fragile, and I just wanted him to be comfortable. It was so reassuring to not see him in pain all the time like I had imagined he would be.

The aftercare went surprisingly well with little to do but keep the stitches dry and clean. It helped so much that Cole was so brave and strong. He never really cried, so one of the hardest things for me was trying to feel content in controlling his pain level. I remember at first not wanting to put him down and once he was down not wanting to pick him up in fear of putting his little body in a hurtful position. Within a short amount of time though, you would never have known that he had major surgery. I learn so much from him every day and can only pray that I can be as strong and resilient to things that come my way as he has.

And he took the children in his arms, put his hands on them and blessed them.

Mark 10:16

I will not leave you comfortless: I will come to you.

John 14:18 KJV

Miles between Us

Still physically and emotionally exhausted from the reflux surgery, Cole and I flew to Arizona for another glaucoma surgery on July 8, 1995. This glaucoma surgery was two hours long, but compared to the reflux surgery, it was fairly routine.

In all, Cole and I bounced back and forth from North Dakota to Arizona for six months. Most of that time was spent in Arizona away from my home and husband. I never imagined Cole and I would be in Arizona so long, but doctor visits and surgeries just kept coming up. During that time, I felt like I was an emotional zombie. There was no time for my emotions to catch up with me. I had to just keep putting one foot in front of the other, always ending up in the same nightmare.

When Cole and I were in Arizona and not rushing in and out of the hospital, we were alone in my parents' house. My dad and mom worked all day, so even though I was staying with family, I felt isolated. I was supposed to be experiencing all the joys of a new family with my husband, but I could not. I did not talk a lot to Mike or any of my friends because we could not afford the phone calls. Sometimes the worry about the medical bills that were piling up was just too much to bear. I would sit on the couch, holding Cole, thinking about how hard Mike and I had worked on his nursery back home. Cole could not see the clowns we had painted on the walls just for him. The dresser that was passed down to him from Mike's family sat empty.

I looked down at my sleeping baby, knowing I could not show him off to my family and friends back in North Dakota. At bath time, I longed for the days when Mike and I would bathe him together.

In my state of loneliness, I began to pray differently than I had before. The prayers that I had come to know and love so well as a child, which gave me great peace, like the Our Father and Hail Mary, suddenly became so impersonal. So I started to talk to God out loud just to keep myself sane. I started to tell him all my fears, hopes, frustrations, and dreams. I asked him what kind of things I should be doing to help Cole get better faster. I asked him to forgive me for all the things I had done wrong and would do wrong. It was then, in my deepest despair while talking with him, that God gave me strength. I did not know it, but it was the beginning of a deep and real relationship with him. I came to realize that my relationship with God would not be recited prayers but actually a one-on-one relationship of us talking to each other.

After Cole's last eye surgery, things started to settle down for a while. We were able to enjoy the rest of the summer without another trip to Arizona. Cole was able to spend a lot of time outside, which we all loved. I was finally seeing a glimpse of what I had always dreamed being a mom was going to be like. It was so refreshing to see Cole play in the grass and start to experience life like every other child does. In November, he was hospitalized for pneumonia again, but other than that, Cole was in pretty good health.

On January 13, 1996, we celebrated Cole's first birthday. He had been through a lot his first year of life, yet he was growing, playing, and being your typical one-year-old. I was amazed at the great strength of this little man. On that day, the day we celebrated the birth of our son, I was filled with complete joy.

Cole was not one year old very long before we had to fly out to Arizona for another surgery. The time had come for his first hypospadias surgery. I could not believe the time had gone so fast. I remember when the doctor told me that they could not circumcise Cole, as they would need to use that skin when he was one to do all the repairs necessary. The surgery Cole would have was four hours long. I was not as scared about this one as I had been during some of the others, but I was angry. I was angry at the situation, and I was angry at God for allowing it. I was angry that Cole had to suffer through yet another surgery. How much more did he have to go through? I felt as if it was going to start all over again. I was in Arizona, away from my husband yet again, wondering when all this would stop. All I wanted and prayed for was to be a normal family, playing in the yard together again.

Managing Cole after the surgery was a challenge as well. He had to keep a catheter in, and it was not easy to keep this very active boy settled down enough to not disturb it. My parents and I came up with different ways to keep him comfortable so we could still give him stroller rides. When the catheter was removed five days later, we were able to go home. A prayer finally answered.

The second part of Cole's hypospadias surgery would not be for another six and a half months. During that time he remained tumor free, his cataract was not getting any bigger, and the glaucoma was staying in control. I felt like I was on a roller coaster, and at that time, I was on the level section of the tracks, just enjoying the ride of getting to know my son. It was so revitalizing to see him crawl, play, and finger feed himself all in the comfort of our own home.

Every night Cole would wrestle with his dad and take a few steps on his own. I did not mind one bit that Cole had to sleep with us most nights, as I think he was having bad dreams with all he had been through so far in his little lifetime. The bed might have been crowded, but at least we were home and together. I also used that time to call other families with aniridia to try to get some suggestions as to what had helped them in my situation. I was determined to be the best mom I could be, to know everything I could, and to give Cole as many opportunities as any child would have growing up. I put Cole on prayer lists and was amazed that people we did not even know placed him on prayer lists as well.

Cole was legally blind, but he was able to see color and shadows at this time in his life. I called a doctor that made special glasses because I had decided to never give up on finding all the things that would make his vision and life better. With the glasses he got, his vision was 20/800 in one eye and 20/600 in the other.

Cole continued to grow up quickly. He started talking and walking and drinking from a cup. He loved swimming, tractor rides, and getting into mischief. All of this I was thankful for along with the fact that he gave the best kisses ever! I thought of the many days when I did not know if any of this would be possible, and I remembered the fear I had that Cole would not be able to enjoy life as he did now.

Rejoice in the Lord always. I will say it again: Rejoice! Let your gentleness be evident to all. The Lord is near. Do not be anxious abut anything, but in everything, by prayer and petition, with thanksgiving, present your requests to God. And the peace of God, which transcends all under standing, will guard your hearts and your minds in Christ Jesus.

Philippians 4:4–7

A Miracle

The summer went by quickly, and fall was upon us. In September, we were devastated once again. Two spots had been found on Cole's left kidney and one on his right kidney. The dreaded Wilms tumor that we never wanted to find was here. This was the hardest thing to deal with, I felt, so far. After such a free and hope-filled summer, here we were again in the hospital, facing the worst once more. I could not help but to think that this would be the end; this time I would be losing him to the great killer, cancer.

I felt every emotion—pain, anger, fear, and even ... peace. This last feeling took me by surprise, as if for a minute a glorious picture of Cole in heaven came into my thoughts. I saw him playing and running like all little boys are supposed to, never again to feel the pain of being cut, poked, or scanned.

That minute of peace ended as quickly as it came. It was replaced with thoughts of never again holding his warm body in my arms, not being able to smell his hair or touch his toes. An ache appeared deep down in my soul feeling like the twisting of a knife. I wanted to grab Cole and run. I wanted to go where no one could take him out of my arms, not even for a second, but I was stuck in that hospital, facing my fears once more.

Mike and I could not comfort each other. There was nothing left in us and therefore nothing to give. We made good medical choices, decisions about surgery, chemo, and medical devices that would be best for our boy; but we could not share with each other our feelings. The grief was too great, the wound too raw.

I do not know how Mike got through it or whom he may have talked to, but as for me, I talked to God and God alone. I did not tell others what I was feeling. I felt the need to be seen as strong and in control. I did not want anyone to see me falter for fear I would be accused of looking for sympathy when I knew how many others were hurting as well. I even felt that because I was no longer working I did not have the right to fall apart. As if not having the stress of holding down a job should somehow minimize what I was going through.

We flew once again to Arizona where the tumors were revealed to us on X-rays and ultrasounds. The tumors were right there, staring us in the face, almost taunting us. Was this really happening? Could it all be a bad dream?

We had heard about a Catholic church that had a healing service scheduled before we had to take Cole in for surgery. We attended that service and took Cole to the front of the church for prayer. The priest placed his hands on Cole, and some of the elders of that church placed their hands on the priest. They then asked the congregation to pray as well. The whole room was filled with prayer, everybody praying in their own way and all for Cole. It felt like that service was just for us, and what a miracle God had given us by placing all the people in our path that would lead up to that wonderful night. Before we left that night we were given holy water and saint medals by people we had never met. It was obvious that these people were genuinely concerned for us and our Cole.

They helped us get through those frightful days before surgery emotionally and spiritually. Just to know that so many were lifting Cole up in prayer meant so much. It gave me a peace that I can only explain as the presence of God through each and every one of them. Even though I was far away from my friends, I felt cared for, and for the first time in a long time, I did not feel like a stranger in a strange town.

The day of the surgery arrived. I had never seen Cole sleep so hard in all his life. He slept through everything! He slept during the entire ride to the hospital. He slept through the changing of his Pull-Ups, the putting in of his IV, and through the whole routine of getting ready to go into surgery.

The nurse that came to get him was a big man, and I will never forget how tiny Cole looked with that nurse holding him. Cole lifted his head up just a little and smiled before he was taken away from us. Just another little way God was showing his presence through it all. The doctor explained to us that the surgery would be at least five to six hours long, but doctors and nurses would be coming out periodically to let us know how it was going.

So once again, we sat—Mike, his parents, me, and my parents. Both Mike's mom and mine had gone down to the cafeteria to get something to drink when the doctor came out for the first time. He walked into the waiting room and placed some X-rays on the table before us. I assumed the worst, and my heart felt as if it had stopped beating. A wave of nausea struck me. I thought I was going to be sick—until I saw the grin spreading across the doctor's face. "I can't explain it," he said. "But the one tumor on the left kidney is gone, and the one on the right is a non-cancerous cyst."

The room exploded with cries and shouts of joy. We couldn't hug each other tight enough! *A miracle at last!* Sweet relief, unexpected, but welcomed in our long, tiring journey.

I ran to tell the grandmas the wondrous news. They saw me running and crying and feared the worst. When I got close enough, I blurted out the great news, and they too were caught up in the wave of joy as tears of happiness flowed in the middle of strong embraces.

Interestingly, during this operation, Cole was cut open from side to side, so when we saw this incision for the first time and how it lay across the scar from the incision from his reflux surgery, it looked like he had a cross on his stomach. Just another sign God was with us.

We were able to attend a Sunday service in the same church where we were prayed over during the healing Mass. The priest recognized us as soon as he saw us. We were thrilled to be able to share in person the miracle that had just occurred. He was so pleased to hear the good news that he picked up Cole, lifted him high for all to see, and marched up to the front of the church where he shared with his entire congregation Cole's miracle. After the service, many came up to look at and touch Cole. I heard several who had walked by praise God for answering this prayer. I marveled at how my boy, so little and modest, was able to share the wonders of God with so many.

Once home again, we continued to share Cole's miracle with others. As we did, God revealed through friends something we had missed. The day of his surgery, when Cole was sleeping so hard, must have been when God was healing him. All of a sudden it all made sense. I needed that miracle. It gave me a renewed strength, and I felt God was showing us that we would make it through anything. I also knew Cole's miracle had touched so many and drew others closer to God. This made it all worth it, not the pain Cole endured, but the miracle God gave us that demonstrated his glory so that others might believe. I felt unbelievably blessed, and my relationship with God moved to a deeper and stronger level. When God touches you in the way he did us, it is a feeling you cannot put into words.

Is any one of you in trouble? He should pray. Is anyone happy? Let him sing songs of praise. Is any one of you sick? He should call the elders of the church to pray over him and anoint him with oil in the name of the Lord. And the prayer offered in faith will make the sick person well; the Lord will raise him up.

James 5:13–15

Therefore, since we have so great a cloud of witnesses surrounding us, let us also lay aside every encumbrance, and the sin which so easily entangles us, and let us run with endurance the race that is set before us.

Hebrews 12:1

The Birth of Clay

Despite the hardships that came with parenthood, Mike and I came to the conclusion that our family was not yet complete. Cole was only two years old when I was pregnant again, but even at such a young age, he was excited. He would often talk with his mouth close to my belly so the baby could hear him. Even with the excitement of soon being a big brother, there was already competition for my attention. I remember one time Cole was insisting that I hold him, but my belly was too big and round to allow this to happen. Cole became frustrated and said, "That's it! Baby, move over. I want to hug Mommy!"

Mike and I were excited, but we were nervous as well. We were scared that our second child would have the same problems as Cole, even though no tests we had taken indicated that would be the case. There was also the concern about how we would handle taking care of a baby as well as all the needs that came with Cole's disability, from always making sure things were picked up around the house and not in walkways for Cole to trip over to the constant way of teaching him daily living skills in a hands-on manner. Then there were the ongoing trips to the doctor every three months for ultrasounds along with the frequent eye doctor visits to make sure his glaucoma pressure was stable. So I was extra careful during my second pregnancy. I took every precaution I could think of to keep this baby healthy.

In spite of the worry and concern, I had a very normal pregnancy with no complications; even the birth was uneventful. The only differences between this birth and Cole's were that my water had to be broken so I would go into labor and there were a lot more doctors waiting around to check the baby out once he had been delivered.

On August 7, 1997, Clay Samuel Roberts was born. As we received all of his statistics and compared them to Cole's, we were amazed to see that the two brothers were always set apart by the number two. Clay was born at 3:33 p.m., and Cole was born at 5:33 p.m.—two hours difference. Clay was twenty-one inches long, and Cole was nineteen inches long—two inches difference. Clay was eight pounds and seven ounces, and Cole was six pounds and seven ounces— two pounds difference. Clay's head was sixteen inches around (ouch!), and Cole's head was fourteen inches around—again, two inches difference.

I held Clay those first few hours and days and found it to be bittersweet. I would look into his big, blue, healthy eyes and be filled with peace and thankfulness. Yet at the same time, I was saddened for Cole and his inability to see the world God has created with all its beauty the way that Clay would be able to.

I had so many mixed emotions on how Cole would be able to interact with his baby brother. I was so sad that he could not see him very well, but as soon as Cole crawled up onto my lap to hold his brother, great contentment came over me as I watched Cole get ever so close to his brother's face and look him over from head to toe. Then he ever so gently kissed his brother's check and said, "I love you, Clay," and with that was off my lap and running to the cabinet in the corner of my hospital room to climb in it once again. At that moment I knew a normal brother relationship had started, and the fears of interaction dissipated. I not only loved every minute I had in the hospital alone with Clay but cherished every minute when the four of us could be on the hospital bed together.

Sons are a heritage from the Lord, children a reward from him.

Psalm 127:3

Worry and Rejection

When Clay was six weeks old, we had to take Cole to the University of Minnesota. This university has a large teaching hospital on its campus. Cole needed surgery on his eye again because his glaucoma was very high and he was in a lot of pain. We had given him medication for the pain, but it didn't relieve him entirely, and I hated to see him hurting so much. About an hour after we had started the drive, I prayed that God would have Cole just fall asleep so he would be unaware of the pain. God answered that prayer, and Cole slept the remaining six hours of this long and nerve-wracking trip.

It was very different having a baby with us as Cole went into surgery. I was unable to focus completely on Cole because I had an infant who needed constant care as well. This was difficult for me because I felt the only thing I could do for Cole was give him my undivided attention when I was with him and my uninterrupted prayers when I was not. I felt this was no longer possible with our new addition to the family.

I found out, however, that it was also a blessing God gave me. Watching over Clay made time go by more quickly, and I did not have time to think about all the *what ifs* while Cole was in surgery. I became content to take care of Clay, while trusting that God was taking care of Cole.

We had plenty of opportunities to perfect juggling a new baby with long trips to Minnesota and sitting in surgery waiting rooms. Cole had three eye surgeries in the first four months of Clay's life. I felt terrible having to drag Clay along on these long trips. To make things worse, Clay was losing weight, and his skin became itchy and irritated. The doctors were really concerned about this, as we didn't know the reason for it. Clay was sleeping okay at night, but his itchy hands would be red and sore by morning. It was so hard to see Clay suffer with this pain, while going to the doctor repeatedly was giving us no answers.

So here we were again. I knew something was wrong with my son, I just did not know what. I was angry at God and the world. I was tired of watching Cole go through surgery after surgery and still have pain. Now Clay was sick and taking test after test to figure out what was causing the rashes. My local doctor took a lot of blood samples with the hope that it would explain what was going on. Unfortunately, she did not get any answers, so she had me trying every cream she could think of, both prescription and over the counter, to try to give Clay some relief. She also took stool samples to try to figure out what was causing the weight loss with no luck.

I was so frustrated at seeing Clay have to go through all the discomfort of his hands along with the needle pokes that were giving no answers on how to make it stop. I was tired of sticking both my boys in the car for seven-hour drives to the hospital and doctor visits. I tried to stay focused on my faith and not get so angry, but I was also physically exhausted from lack of sleep. All I wanted was to see my boys playing the way they were supposed to.

Just when my thoughts were at their darkest and I thought I could take no more, I would see my boys smiling. Clay would laugh and Cole would pray, and that gave me a little more strength to keep going. I would remember how blessed I was just to have them both, and I was thankful because I knew things could be worse.

By this time, I had begun searching for a support group. I wanted to share things I had learned and learn things I did not know. I found one that was based out of town. They sent out newsletters that had helpful information about WAGR, as well as stories of those afflicted with it. I had received their newsletter and talked to a few of its members. Then I got a phone call I did not expect, which hurt so deeply. I was asked to not participate much in this group. Although Cole had his hardships dealing with WAGR, he apparently did not have some of the same hardships as the other children with the same affliction. Cole had the Wilms tumor, aniridia, and genital defects, but never had the mental retardation. I prayed this did not seem shallow or uncaring, but in my thoughts I was thankful for this. I was told that if I spoke too much about how well Cole was doing I could make the other families feel bad.

At first I was confused. To me, being a part of this group was like being in the house of the Lord. In God's house, you can feel connected to all who are present because you have something in common—Christ. It does not matter where you are on your journey with him. Some may be just starting their walk. Some may have been on the journey of a lifetime and have a deep, powerful relationship, and then there are all of us in between. It doesn't matter, because everyone is learning and growing from each other, no matter where they are in their walk.

I thought it should be the same with this group. We had WAGR in common. Some had it more severe than others, but I felt that we could all grow and learn from each other. I felt lost when I was asked to not speak too much about the good things Cole was doing. To me, that did not make sense because bad and good so often go together. I had a strong passion to learn and not just sit around, read stories, and feel sorry for myself. I thought I had finally found a group of people in similar situations as me, a group with commonalities that could understand the pain and hardship I was going through, only to be told Cole and I were not suffering enough to earn their support. I was in no man's land.

God is good and I was not left empty-handed. I still keep in touch with a wonderful lady from that group who has helped me out so much with advice on doctors and questions I have about WAGR.

As I write this, I realize it was a blessing to not be a part of that support group. With all the pain and fear of the unknown I was dealing with, I am sure I would have relied too heavily on others, when I needed to rely fully on God. Through this, I feel God has helped me see the blessing for my family. God has also shown me that my support group is his house and my supporters are both himself and his people. He has told me so in his own words in the Bible.

Praise be to the God and Father of our Lord Jesus Christ, the Father of compassion and the God of all comfort, who comforts us in all our troubles, so that we can comfort those in any trouble with the comfort we ourselves have received from God. For just as the sufferings of Christ flow over into our lives, so also through Christ our comfort overflows.

2 Corinthians 1:3–5

Fighting for Sight

Within just a few months, Cole had seven surgeries on his left eye in an effort to keep it from dying. It was getting to the point where every time we would get into the car he would become distressed and ask if we were going to the hospital for another surgery. This really shook me up as I got a glimpse at what all this was doing to him emotionally. Imagine being afraid every time you had to go in the car!

We talked to the doctor and did a lot of research. We found out that if we continued with the eye surgeries there was only a 5 percent chance they would make any difference. Even if those surgeries did succeed, we would have to do many more of them just to keep his eye working. Armed with this information, we prayed and talked to Cole about what to do. We decided that for the sake of our son's emotional health the eye surgeries would need to stop.

Mike and I grieved for the loss of the eye that we felt we were giving up on, but when we told Cole there would be no more eye surgeries, he jumped up and down and yelled with excitement. When the eye pressure gets too low in an eye, the eye dies; and it can either die painfully, which results in the eye having to be removed, or it can die quietly. Praise God, Cole's eye died quietly, and we did not have to remove it. Cole adjusted very well, and we began to see his emotions improve significantly. It was a relief to see him get into the car without any fear. Even with

Cole's positive outlook, I was not so optimistic. Anger toward God was renewed, as well as self-doubt. I wondered if I could have prayed harder or more often, or maybe I wasn't a good enough Christian for God to take my prayers seriously. Overall, the same question still hung over my head as it had since Cole was first diagnosed—*why?*

That same summer, the summer of 1998, we also had concerns for Clay. He seemed to always be sick with stomachaches, and he had developed an awful rash on his entire body. We found ourselves once again marching from one doctor to the next to pinpoint what was going on with him. We were getting extremely nervous because he was still losing so much weight.

My doctor did more blood tests, which only led to more frustration, medical bills, and no answers. With nothing left to do, she sent me to a local dermatologist who was worried that Clay had a rare skin disorder because of the way the rash looked. In her office she took a skin sample from Clay's back. You would think I would be able to tolerate this, but it was really hard for me to see him go through this. He cried so hard, and it took the doctor and two nurses to hold him down. After they were done, I just felt sick to my stomach as I held his sweaty little body close to me while we waited for the results. I remember getting so mad when the doctor came in and told me that the skin they took just looked like eczema under the microscope and sent me home with another new cream to try.

It felt like I was getting on the same roller coaster that I swore I would never go on again. Have you ever done that? You go on a ride that is so terrifying you absolutely hate every minute of it. A few months later, the carnival comes back to town, and what do you do? Yup! Get right back on that same ride. You just start to move, and fear kicks in, your heart races, and you say to yourself, "No! I did not want to do this again!" But it is too late. You no longer have any control over stopping and getting off.

That is what I felt like when we could not find out what was wrong with Clay. I was worried I would not have the energy or faith to do it all over again. I felt self-pity knocking at my door along with thoughts of *why me again?* I did the only thing I could and took my burdens to God. I prayed he would get me off this roller coaster and if that was not to be done that he would help me find joy in this terrifying ride. Finally I prayed, "Please ride with me, God. Help me to not fall out."

We had to travel to the University of Minnesota to find our answers for Clay. The doctors performed allergy tests on him, a lot of them! It turned out that he is allergic to many things, such as peanuts, milk, soy, peas, wheat, and corn. We were faced with the new challenge of how to feed our son without making him sick. At least now we knew what we were dealing with. I kept Clay away from all the things he could not have and lathered him in a steroid cream for about a month. His skin cleared up so nicely. It was like he was a totally different little boy.

The concern I had on what to feed him quickly left, as I was able to find the rice milk at my local grocery store along with some foods he loved like potatoes cut in squares and either fried or boiled. I was so happy to have Clay feeling better and looking better that the high cost of his rice milk did not even matter to me. It was challenging to find a healthy diet with variety at a reasonable cost, but I did my best to make it work. One night as I was praying, God implanted in my brain, "You cannot put a price tag on a healthy son." So at that moment I still had uneasiness financially but knew deep down God would provide.

Whatever difficulties my boys had—Cole now three and Clay one year—it didn't stop them from being boys. There was no way I was going to hold them back from doing what they wanted to do and should do as children. We went to the zoo twelve times that summer. I had to give Clay Benadryl and a medicated breathing treatment before going, and sometimes I would give him the treatment during and after the zoo visits as well. We also swam a lot; both boys loved the water. Mike and I would ride our bikes, pulling the boys behind in a bike cart, and Cole and Mike would sleep outside in the tent.

As a mom I loved how well the boys got along with each other. Sure, there was the occasional pushing or hitting, as brothers will do, but it was obvious they loved each other very much. Before I knew it, Cole was old enough to graduate from the home visits we were getting weekly with an early intervention teacher to work on life skills with his low vision to now being old enough for his first day of preschool. He went to the school that his early intervention teacher worked at, which was a school for children with disabilities. This was great because this school had special services available that would help him prepare for reading Braille, as well as other programs that would meet his specific needs.

Cole still had some sight in one eye, so teaching him Braille was an option, but something told us we should go ahead and do it. This was a much harder decision than I thought it would be. I had to make myself go to a place I rarely went, the place of accepting that Cole some day could be completely blind.

Cole blended in with the rest of the school kids very well, almost too well. He immersed himself into the classes and his new friends. It was hard to see this in the sense that I thought he would miss me too much to want to interact with them. I would have felt better if he missed his mommy a little more than he did. I think maybe all moms feel that way about their children's first days away from home.

Cole loved school, and he definitely wasn't shy. He sang songs and answered questions starting that very first day. I realized I stayed in the classroom that first day not for Cole's sake but for my own. That afternoon when we got home, Cole had so much to tell his dad, and Clay had so much to tell me, as he got to stay home and play with his dad. We were all so excited about our day that we did not want it to end, so Cole and I took Clay and Dad to the school to play on Cole's new playground. This also gave me a chance to show Clay what it was like just in case we needed to stay some days at the school, when Mike had to be at work.

That year, Cole was enrolled in Kinder Music, a program that uses music to teach young children basic rhythms as well as encouraging the enjoyment of music. He also took swimming lessons. He enjoyed all these things, but I think I took greater pleasure in his participation because it showed me and the rest of the world that Cole was not letting his disability slow him down one bit.

He said to them, "Let the little children come to me, and do not hinder them, for the kingdom of God belongs to such as these."

Mark 10:14

Though he brings grief, he will show compassion, so great is his unfailing love. For he does not willingly bring affliction or grief to the children of men.

Lamentations 3:32–33

A Visit to Heaven

At this time, things were going pretty well, which made me a little nervous. I worried that this was the calm before a large storm. I don't know if I will ever be able to enjoy the tranquil times of life again without that thought entering my mind. We were getting better at figuring out Clay's diet, Cole's ultrasounds were coming back clear, and the year went by with only the typical ups and downs—and by *typical* I mean typical for energetic little boys.

It was startling to me how quickly I could lose sight of God's presence when all was going well. You would think that this would be the time I felt him the most, but my humanness of wanting to be in control and self-sufficient was too great. As I look back and reflect on this time, I can honestly say that my prayer life had greatly diminished.

I remember one Sunday, Clay, Mike, and I were supervising the nursery at church, and Clay discovered the "sit-n-spin." Only, Clay decided to stand-n-spin. This did not work well, and he ended up falling off and cutting himself above the eye, which would need five stitches. This was not one of my better moments. You would think that with all the surgeries and other things we had been through I would have stayed very calm. Unfortunately, this was not the case. As I scooped Clay up, my all white outfit was quickly covered in blood. I carried him through the church, frantically looking for someone to take over the nursery. I still wonder what people thought as they saw me carrying this little boy, both of us covered in blood, yelling, "We have had a little accident; can someone take over in the nursery?" When we got to the ER, Clay was so brave; he did not cry at all as the doctor put in five stitches above his eye. Once home and everyone was settled in, Mike and I laughed as we debated if the church would let us work the nursery again.

Another time, I was baking, and Clay reached into the oven to investigate the "pretty red things." I could not get to him in time, and he ended up burning his hand. The burn was bad enough for a trip to the doctor, who wrapped up his little hand and gave us medication for it. It was surprisingly quick how all of a sudden I was not in control and needed, or should I say wanted, and begged for God's help with the well-being of my child. At the moment my prayer life went into overdrive. When all was finished and Clay was taken care of, I decided to get Cole a flu shot. The next day he was so sick that the doctor suggested we never give him a flu shot again. So I had at home with me one small boy, extremely sick, and another even smaller boy with a pained hand.

Still another time, Cole and Clay were having a blast jumping on the bed. Cole fell and landed on his arm. He cried for only a moment, so I assumed he had only bruised it a little. Seven days later when Cole was still not bending his arm, I decided to have it checked out by a doctor, who promptly put Cole's broken arm into a cast.

It wasn't long after Cole had the cast taken off when he fell again and said that his arm was hurting. We knew the drill and what came next. We rushed him to the clinic, and sure enough, every time the doctor would touch his arm, he would say "ouch" and cry. X-rays were taken, but there was no sign of a break or even a sprain; but the doctor took his cue from Cole's behavior and put his arm in a sling.

As we left, Mike and I were emotionally drained. Our minds were filled with what others might think about Cole constantly getting hurt when suddenly Cole lifted up his "hurt" arm and triumphantly stated, "All right! More stickers!" The minute the words left his lips, he knew he had made a serious mistake and froze. He was done, caught, or should I say busted. All he wanted was more stickers, and in his young mind, with everything he had been through, you had to be hurt or sick to get them. His punishment was having to sit through a serious talk about the importance of not faking a sickness or being hurt. As I revisit that moment in my mind, I can't hold back the smile.

There were other surprises as well. One day, Cole had just finished taking a nap when he came downstairs and confronted me. "You lied to me," he accused, in a matter-of-fact tone. I was confused. I couldn't think of when I would have lied to my son. "You told me Bridget was on a farm, but she isn't," Cole continued. "She is in heaven." I couldn't believe my ears. Cole was right; Bridget was our dog, and we had to put her down. We were worried how that might upset Cole and Clay, so we told them we had sent her to a farm with a big yard where she would be able to run around and play. We were so worried about our *story* being blown that we didn't tell *anyone* else a different version. Cole was right; Bridget was in heaven. I asked Cole how he had found out she was in heaven, and what he told me next came as a shock. "I was there, in heaven, and I played with her."

At first I could not believe my ears; did Cole have a dream? But why and how did he know Bridget was put down? This and so many other questions raced through my mind. So I took a deep breath, sat him on my lap, and told him to tell me everything about his dream. Cole went into such astonishing detail of his dream about what he did in heaven with Bridget. They played ball and sat on a cloud as he hugged her. The more Cole talked, this incredible feeling came over me that he was telling the truth, and I felt God telling me to believe. I thought instantly of the verse "Let the little children come to me, and do not hinder them, for the kingdom of God belongs to such as these" (Mark 10:14 NIV).

Later, when Mike came home, we questioned him about his trip to heaven. He described it again in such detail, more than you would think a boy who could barely see should know. It was pretty simple to Cole; in heaven, he could see just fine. He could see Bridget, the wonderful colors of the fluffy clouds, and the magnificent bright lights that illuminated the sky. I have to admit, I had to fight the human feelings of, *This cannot be true, and I would be crazy to believe this.* Once again, though, the feeling of truth overwhelmed me, and I stopped fighting it and praised God for such a wonderful gift that he had given to Cole. Then I actually for a moment became jealous of this gift, a gift that was so unique. Quickly this passed, and such joy came over me I felt God was showing me Cole will see through him, maybe not on this earth but in heaven and in his timing.

At that time Jesus, full of joy through the Holy Spirit, said, "I praise you, Father, Lord of heaven and earth, because you have hidden these things from the wise and learned, and revealed them to little children. Yes, Father, for this was your good pleasure.

Luke 10:21

How Much More, God!

When Cole was five years old, we had an artificial eye made for him. We had to travel to Fargo, North Dakota, which is about a three-hour drive. Even though he could not see out of his left eye, it was still healthy enough to place a shell-like cover around it. The procedure to make this eye involved a lot of steps, and it took most of a day to do it. The doctor was very kind and even let Cole paint a little of the iris and pupil on his new eye.

When it was finished, it was a little larger than a quarter in size and in thickness. The doctor explained that the care of the shell was very easy; all we needed to do was wash it every time before we put it in. This was to cut down on the risk of getting infections. He showed us how to take it in and out using this special little suction cup-like tool. This part was not as easy because the shell was so big and Cole wanted to automatically close his eye for protection. So the doctor worked with Cole until Cole was able to put it on and take it out by himself.

Cole's natural iris was light gray in color, and the eye itself was exceptionally white and smaller than normal. The human eyelid needs a full-sized eye to open it. Cole was unable to open his eye all the way due to his own eyeball being so small from dying.

With the artificial eye, this was no longer a problem. His eyelid was able to open all the way to show off this new, authentic-looking eye. Cole was very handsome even without his new eye, but with it in, he really looked great. As I looked at Cole with his brand new eye, I couldn't help but marvel at the technology God has given us. I praised God for this, and I thanked him for keeping Cole's eye healthy enough to have this shell placed over it.

Two months later, I noticed that Cole's artificial eye was not in after he had woken up from a nap. I became anxious because that eye had cost $1,200. Cole told me where he had placed it, and I immediately went to get it. It was exactly where Cole said it would be, but it was broken. Cole said it must have broken when he set it down after taking it out. My heart sank, but I told myself these things happen.

We went back to the doctor in Fargo to get another eye made. As he examined the broken eye, we told him what happened, according to what Cole had told us. The doctor started to laugh and said, "I see; is that why there are teeth marks on it?"

Cole was busted! Having been exposed, Cole explained that he just wanted to see what it tasted like. The doctor told us that this actually happens a lot. Kids just can't resist trying to eat it. Driving home, I had to laugh because I can honestly say I have never wanted to taste an eyeball! My soul laughed with me as I was blessed to enjoy this part of life through the heart of a child—even at the cost of $1,200.

Cole wore the eye for about eight months. During that time, he would get infections under the shell, and this caused him great pain. He did not think it was worth all the pain that came with it, so he decided to not wear the artificial eye anymore. He knew some people might be uncomfortable when they saw him with his natural eye but decided that those people did not need to look at him then.

I was very proud that Cole had enough confidence in himself to not be concerned with what others thought. At such a young age, he knew life was not about looks, but rather it was about one's character and relationship with God. Again this little boy strengthened my faith without even knowing it because he helped to remind me what is truly important, something at my ripe old age, I still have trouble remembering, especially when I start to worry about material things.

Another year went by in the typical Roberts fashion. Clay had his adenoids taken out to help with his breathing problems and sinus infections. Cole had his adenoids taken out, and he also had tubes put into his ears, two broken arms, and a broken nose. Nothing too major, wouldn't you agree? Cole's adenoids were taken out in hopes to reduce the amount of colds and sinus infections he was getting. He had tubes put in his ears to reduce ear infections. He broke one arm simply falling just right while at play. He broke the second arm falling out of a hammock that he and Clay had been wrestling in. Immediately after the cast had been taken off of his arm, he broke his nose when he was playing in the back of our pickup truck and fell out. We were beginning to get a little worried that the doctors would call social services to investigate us. My prayer for Cole had always been that he would be able to act like every other boy his age. I added to that prayer an additional request—that he would also be more careful, because even though he could hardly see, that boy had no fear.

Again, the surprises of all these physical events were not without surprises of a spiritual nature. After waking up one morning, Cole again mentioned that he had gone to heaven, and this time he met Jesus. He did not talk a lot about it; he simply said it was special. It took everything I had in me not to want to ask Cole questions about this new adventure he was so blessed in getting to partake in. I do not know about you, but I have dreamed of seeing Jesus face to face, and here my son was telling me he had. I felt so overwhelmed with great awe that God would bless Cole yet again with another gift from heaven. I really believe God was giving Cole this to help prepare him for the great journey that he has laid before him. All I could do was keep saying over and over in my head, *Thank you, Jesus.*

Cole was by this time a kindergartener. He went to a public school where he would have to learn his ABCs both in writing and in Braille. He loved the work, and he loved being with all the kids. He hated missing school, and he almost always came home happy and with lots and lots to say. This gave me great peace as I knew God again answered a prayer that I had prayed when Cole was first diagnosed with aniridia. I remember thinking that he would never go to school, never have friends, and never be able to do anything without me. God was showing me differently!

Clay was actually going to the same preschool for disabled children that Cole had gone to. He was asked to be a model student there. A model student is one who is not disabled but can model for the other children how to do everyday tasks with appropriate social interaction. I worked there that year as an aid so I could be with Clay. He loved going to the same school that his big brother had gone to, and he felt so big when he rode the bus home, even though it was only for a short time, and I was driving in my car behind them. I remember saying to him, "I will be right behind you; I will never let you out of my sight." I pictured in my mind that day how God must feel when I start to venture out on my own. He wants to give me freedom, but he is also there to protect me at the same time.

Surely God is my salvation; I will trust and not be afraid. The Lord, the Lord, is my strength and my song; he has become my salvation. With joy you will draw water from the wells of salvation.

Isaiah 12:2–3

The Car Accident

We had never given up on finding a doctor that might know how to give Cole his sight. I would clip articles and look for eye specialists all over the world. When I would find one, I would send them Cole's information to see if they could help my precious son.

In my research, I ran across the name of a doctor in Ohio who was the first to do stem cell transplants in the eye that would help cornea transplants be more effective. When Cole's eye died, his cornea got cloudy, so I made an appointment to see this specialist.

In December, we went down to Cincinnati, Ohio. It turned out that Cole needed a new cornea. We went back home with lots to read and began the process of deciding what all needed to be done to get him that new cornea.

Next, we had to travel to Minneapolis to see a retina specialist. There, we discussed what should be done to prepare Cole's eye for the cornea transplant. At this time, Cole's glaucoma was being controlled by drops, but this visit told us that Cole would need a tube-shunt put in, just like the other eye had. There was so much scar tissue built up from all the surgeries on the drainage angle of Cole's eye that something more aggressive was necessary. The tube-shunt procedure would place a tube in his eye to do the draining for the normal drainage system.

While driving back to North Dakota, the weather turned bad. Snow and sleet made driving hazardous and slow. We called home to say we would be late and found out that Clay, who stayed behind on this trip, was in the ER. He had been riding in the car with Mike's dad when another car ran a red light and hit them. I could not get a hold of him right away, and my thoughts turned to the worst. I had this picture of Clay hurt really badly and afraid.

When we got a hold of Mike's mom, she told us he was fine and was at home with them, resting. She pleaded with us to drive carefully and to not worry. Even though we heard her words, Mike and I could not stop feeling troubled. We felt guilty and angry. We couldn't help but to think that if not for all these doctor appointments our family could just be together. Cole would not have to get ready for surgeries, and Clay would not be hurt. I was mad, scared, and frustrated all at the same time.

The weather and worry weighed heavily on the rest of the trip home, which seemed to take an eternity. Our minds were on Clay, and yet at the same time, Cole was in the backseat, tired from sitting in the car for so long. My mind did a crazy dance of jumping from Cole and what the next step in his journey was, to Clay, who was so far from me and who I could not get to fast enough. I started to pray, "God, please keep him safe, please do not let anything be wrong, and please comfort him if he is scared and in pain." I was tired, the road was perilous, and the car seemed to want to crawl along ever so slowly.

My mind kept wandering into that area where our worst thoughts hide. *What will he look like? Could I have stopped it if I was home? Why did I leave him? Is he going to die? This is my fault; I am a terrible mom.* When we finally made it home, I saw Clay without a cut or scratch on him. I touched him, held him, and only then could I free myself from those terrible and tormenting thoughts.

The next day, we went to see the car. I was amazed that Clay had not been seriously injured because he was sitting on the side of the car that was hit. Clay had fallen asleep, so he was already lying down. This was a blessing because the impact did not jar him as hard or throw him down; however, he was covered with glass from the shattered window and was taken to the ER just to make sure that no pieces of glass went into his eyes or skin. Back at Grandma and Grandpa's house, they tried in vain to pick all the glass out of Clay's hair and clothes until finally Grandma Mary took out the vacuum and vacuumed him from head to toe.

As I looked at the car and saw what *could* have happened to Clay and Grandpa, and then realized what little actually *did* happen, another thought came to my mind that was both disturbing and comforting. I realized that I needed to be with both boys, but that was not humanly possible. Then I realized that only God could truly keep them both safe. I think the hardest thing a mother can do is completely trust her children to the unseen hands of God. Yet when we do, and sometimes it's not by choice, we can see the work those hands have done and will continue to do because of his unending love for us.

We are glad whenever we are weak but you are strong; and our prayer is for your perfection.

2 Corinthians 13:9

But let all who take refuge in you be glad; let them ever sing for joy. Spread your protection over them, that those who love your name may rejoice in you.

Psalm 5:11

Surgery Yet Again

My mom and dad had left Arizona and moved back to North Dakota. Mom graciously watched Cole for me one day. After I picked him up and took him home, she called me to let me know that Cole had told her he had met her brother.

My mom had two brothers. One is alive and well, but the other had passed away. I was very young when this happened, and we have never talked much about him. In fact, the very nature of his death to this day is not very clear to me. Naturally, my mom assumed Cole meant he had met her living brother. She agreed with him, "Yes, honey, I know you have met your uncle when he came to visit." Cole, come to find out, did not mean the uncle he had met here on Earth. He was talking about the uncle he met in heaven. He knew his uncle's name, despite the fact that we never talked about him. He knew what he looked like, despite the fact he had never seen a picture of him. In fact, there are no pictures of him displayed in anybody's house. His pictures are kept in old photo albums, and even if we would have tried to show Cole a picture of him, Cole has never had good enough vision to be able to see one clearly.

We did not ask Cole much about this trip to heaven. We did not want to make his trips into a big deal; however, in my heart and thoughts, I was yearning for this gift that Cole had received from God. We were afraid that if we revealed our fascination on the subject he might be prone to make things up, as little kids often do in search for more attention. We wanted to be sure that each experience he had would remain real and true. Each trip was a special gift from God just for Cole, and we did not want to diminish it in any way. This gift that he was so kindly given not only renewed but also reinforced my faith and trust in God's unending love and grace for my family. It kindled a yearning deep in my soul to live my life for him in a richer way every day not for my glory but his alone.

The day after Christmas, Cole's right eye started to bleed inside because his retina had detached. We jumped into the car and raced to Minnesota. God was at the wheel, because we made the trip in five hours instead of the usual seven. Once there, Cole's glaucoma specialist and retina specialist performed emergency surgery on his eye. Surgery went well, and we came home soon after. Two weeks later, his retina came off again, so we made another trip to Minnesota for another emergency surgery.

As sick as I was with having to deal with more unexpected surgeries, I was even sicker at the thought of Cole losing what sight he still had. At this time, he could only see light and some shadows. He could no longer see well enough to read or see things close up. Both Cole and I were dealing with the loss of his sight, and we were both angry.

Cole's anger came out in ways of communication, never behavioral. For such a young boy, he handled his anger in a very grown-up matter. He would talk to me about how mad he was with God and ask what I thought were very appropriate questions like, "When will the surgeries stop? Why me? Why will God not answer my prayers?" I had no answers for him except to keep praying and not give up hope. This was so hard because he would answer with, "Why pray, Mom?" He was not hearing me, but because I myself was dealing with the same anger and the same questions. I do not know why I blamed God because I knew deep down he loved Cole and did not want to see him suffer. The only explanation I could come up with was that I had no one else I could blame.

That January 2002 was the start of a very long and hard road. Cole had just turned seven, and he was constantly undergoing eye surgery after eye surgery. It would seem like we would just get home when we would have to turn around and go back again. Some of his surgeries were planned, but others were not. We would drive like crazy and pull into the ER, where they would take him from us and wheel him straight into surgery.

I did not want to give up, but at the same time, somewhere so deep down in a place I rarely ever let myself go, I knew he would lose the fight that he was so bravely fighting. I looked out of the hospital room window, and in the park across the street, I saw prostitutes and drug dealers in plain sight. I kept asking God why. Why would he take sight from this sweet little boy while these people moved about, free to destroy their lives and the lives of others?

A thought flashed through my mind: *There must not be a God, so why bother to do what's good?* Then faith, like a strong wind, shoved that thought out of my mind, and I knew God was there. I can't explain how I knew; I just did.

During every surgery, a gas bubble was placed in Cole's eye to hold his retina in place. After every surgery, Cole would have to keep his head down so the bubble would stay at the back of the eye to push against his retina. He would even have to sleep with his little head down. He always did a wonderful job at keeping his head down, and never did he complain. The whole time, he remained very positive and very courageous.

Clay was also very good during this time. Most of his life, he knew that if I was on the phone and packing, a trip was only minutes away. He sat through many long hours of car rides to and from Minnesota, and he always found something to do in the boring waiting rooms. I knew these trips must have been very tedious for a five-year-old boy, but he always chose to go with us. He never wanted to stay with anybody else when we had to leave. I feel that God put it in his heart to want to go along with us on these lengthy and stressful trips because otherwise we would not have been together very much. I feel that because of Clay's desire to always come along our family remained together and became stronger in the end.

Cast your cares on the Lord and he will sustain you; he will never let the righteous fall. But you, O God, will bring down the wicked into the pit of corruption; bloodthirsty and deceitful men will not live out half their days. But as for me, I trust in you.

Psalm 55:22

Trust in the Lord with all your heart, and lean not unto your own understanding. In all your ways acknowledge him. And he will direct your paths.

Proverbs 3:5–6

Angels in the Midst of Blindness

My sister-in-law, Laura, headed up a breakfast benefit and silent auction for Cole. It was such a blessing. So many people showed up to help us out and honor Cole. No one would let me do any of the work, even though I would have loved to help all those who were working so hard to make this benefit a success. Instead, I got the great privilege to talk with those who attended. I watched as people came up to the message board that spoke of Cole's life with pictures and stories. I joined them in their tears as they read about Cole's struggles and all the surgeries he had already been through at his young age. I was surrounded by kind and loving people who genuinely cared for us. I felt God in the midst of all this. Somehow, his presence is magnified when we all gather together to help one another. I felt so unworthy and prayed that the other benefits scheduled for that same day would be as prosperous.

Cole was only there for a short time. He was very sore and tired from his most recent surgery. His cousin Matt had taken him to the bathroom and in his eagerness to help Cole had perhaps underestimated Cole's abilities to pretty much take care of himself. Cole, in his fatigue, became frustrated, turned to his cousin, and said, "Matt, I am not blind; I just cannot see!" I will never forget Cole saying those words, as they are absolutely his motto for life.

The surgeries Cole was having on his eye were to prepare him for his cornea transplant. The transplant would not take place for a few months, and in the meantime, Cole could not play or swim. He had to keep his head down all the time, and he was getting tired of it. It was hard to watch Cole live this way, basically unable to do much of anything.

Mike and I decided it was time for a reality check. We knew the cornea transplant could save Cole's eye, but it would also mean many more surgeries just to keep it working, and even then there were no guarantees of success. There was a decision we needed to make. *Do we continue with this struggle to maintain Cole's eye, or do we let the eye go?* We gave this a great deal of thought and prayer before heading down to Minnesota for one more very important eye appointment. This one would tell us which direction we should go.

I can still see what the waiting room looked like. The large sculpture on the office coffee table, lots of books in large print, and many other adults waiting just like we were. The room smelled like coffee as I watched people coming and going in slow motion. Somehow, that scene became frozen in my mind as we waited to decide the fate of what was left of Cole's sight.

We were led into the doctor's examining room. I could not breathe for fear of what the doctor was going to say. I did not trust myself to look at Cole because my emotions were starting to slip out of my control. The doctor came in and got straight to the point. I was surprised to notice that he too was having a difficult time controlling his emotions.

Before he started the examination, Cole had asked if he could say a prayer. Once again, I was amazed at Cole's faith in God at such a young age, and once again, he helped me through his obedience to God. The doctor honored Cole's request to pray, even though he was of a different faith.

After the examination, the doctor asked if we wanted Cole to leave the room while he told us his findings. We felt Cole deserved to hear what the doctor had to say, so he remained in the room. The doctor struggled to tell us the chances were slim that any more surgeries could help save Cole's eye. He turned his back to us and cleared his throat many times before he could get out the words, "There isn't much more we can do."

We all looked at Cole with a great deal of apprehension. The decision to continue trying with surgeries or to stop was his. This little boy, whose biggest decision should be what truck to play with, was now making life-changing choices.

The air in the room was thick with the emotion of loss. Cole sat in the large examination chair surrounded by medical equipment. Mike and I were sitting in the corner, feeling far too far away from him. "Doctor," Cole asked. "If I have no more surgeries, can I wrestle?"

"Yes."

"Do I have to keep my head down anymore?"

"No."

Cole jumped out of his chair, raised his arm in triumph, and yelled, "*Yes, yes, I can wrestle, and no more surgeries!*"

He gave the doctor a big hug and wanted to leave immediately! Cole could have felt sorry for himself, but he did not. At that moment, I watched my little boy, who was in such agony just a few minutes ago, now jumping and smiling. During that triumphant moment, it did not sink in what we would have to deal with when Cole lost complete vision. That moment was not filled with anxiety of the unknown. No, that moment was Cole's, and I rejoiced with him.

On the way home, I noticed Cole was staring out of the window. Cole would look out of the window now and then, but I had never before seen him do it for as long as he did this time. Finally he said, "Mommy, I can see them."

"Who do you see?" I asked.

"The angels … look, Mommy … there! Here they come."

Mike and I thought that maybe he saw or even felt the sun, but Cole insisted on what he saw. "Beautiful blue lights with long, flowing, white dresses, so pretty, Mommy. There are three of them." I didn't know at that time what to think or believe. The doctors would tell us that he would see the heat of light (his brain making the images his eyes could not see anymore) and maybe the light would hit the blood in his eye just right and cause flashes. As I pondered this event, I remembered the miraculous healing he had as a baby and his trips to heaven, and I am convinced that my blind son knew what he was seeing.

This glimpse into a spiritual world that is always around all of us was to give him strength and let him know everything would be okay. He was being encouraged by a quick reminder of the beauty of heavenly things. For me, encouragement would be an understatement. I saw Christ through the breath of my child, and it took me aback. I truly felt that the angels were sent as a constant reminder for me that God is protecting us in the spiritual world, that the guardian angels I heard about and believed in as a child really do exist. Before this moment in my adult life, I could dismiss them, but not anymore.

Walk by faith, not by sight.

2 Corinthians 5:7 KJV

For he will command his angels concerning you to guard you in all your ways.

Psalm 91:11

I have no greater joy than to hear that my children are walking in the truth.

3 John 1:4

Bobby in Heaven

The boys and I attended the funeral of an eight-year-old boy who had sadly lost his battle to cancer. His name was Bobby, and he wrestled on the same team as Clay. Even though he was a few years older than Clay, he would come over to his end of the wrestling mat during practice and teach him different wrestling moves. It wasn't until after wrestling season was over that I had heard people talking about Bobby. He was diagnosed with cancer, and eight months later, he had lost the fight against this uncaring, ugly disease.

The funeral itself was remarkable in the way that it completely and truly honored Bobby's life here on Earth. I saw Doreen, a mother who had to say good-bye to her son, and a wave of thankfulness washed over me. I was thankful for all of the trials we were facing and thankful for the journey we were walking with Cole. For despite the many surgeries and the blindness, I could still touch him. I could still smell that little boy smell as he sat there beside me. I could turn to look at him, and I would be able to see him. I could do all these things sitting in a church behind a woman who would never get that chance again. Yes, I was thankful, but in the midst of that thankfulness, my heart ached for Doreen, and I felt God nudging me to contact her. So I called her, and we started to connect. Cole also felt drawn to her almost immediately. He talked about Doreen and her family a lot and often asked me how she was doing.

One morning, Cole approached me and told me he had gone to heaven and met Bobby there. I listened to the account of his visit to heaven and found it to be very intriguing and remarkable. Then he asked me if he could call Doreen, as he had something to tell her. You could probably imagine my reaction. What a request! Do I let my son call up a woman who had just lost her son to say, "Hey, I just saw your boy in heaven"? Or do I decline and not believe him? Cole persisted, and I prayed…a lot! Finally I agreed to let Cole talk to Doreen. My hands shook as I dialed her number. When she answered, my heart beat wildly, and I tried my best to explain the reason for the call. I told her that Cole had said he went to heaven and played with Bobby, and now he wanted to talk to her. I found myself apologizing over and over and saying I hoped this was not hurting her.

Doreen was very kind and graciously said, "Of course I will talk to Cole." I heard Cole's side of the conversation. I heard him tell her that he and Bobby played by jumping from cloud to cloud, and then they just sat and talked. I could tell Doreen was asking questions when I heard Cole answering them. I heard him tell her about a baseball cap and wrestling shoes. When they were finished talking, I took the phone and heard Doreen sobbing on the other end. I felt just horrible. Then, to my astonishment, I heard her say, "Thank you, thank you."

Cole told her things about Bobby that only the family would have known. They had placed Bobby's little cap and wrestling shoes in his casket. Cole knew these things even though Bobby had a closed casket funeral. Doreen believes Bobby did talk to Cole and that Bobby had Cole talk to her so she could know he was all right.

This was not the only time Cole played with Bobby in heaven. It happened three more times. One of those times, they were playing with a rabbit. When Cole told this to Doreen, she revealed that on the last day of Bobby's life on Earth, a rabbit showed up at their back door and did not leave. Even after Bobby passed, a rabbit would show up on days when Doreen felt especially sad or alone.

The fourth time Cole saw Bobby in heaven I knew it would be the last time. Bobby had told Cole to let his mom know he was fine, and now she should take care of his brother, Joe, and sister, Rachel.

Cole did not visit heaven after that; at least, if he did, he did not talk to us about it. What a gift God gave to Cole and to Bobby's family. I know that it was by God's hand our families were brought together because of little things that happened between us. There are too many things to share them all, but I will share my favorite one. I felt led to get Doreen and her family, of all things, a strawberry plant. Not flowers or a card, but a strawberry plant! When we presented it to Doreen, she began to cry. As it turned out, one of the few things Bobby was able to eat his last precious days were strawberries. The little plant produced strawberries that year for Bobby's family, and when a little rabbit showed up, they were happy to let it nibble on its fruit.

Doreen has talked to me many times since of what a great blessing this was for her, as it gave her strength in knowing Bobby was truly taken care of in God's hands. This did not make the pain and hurt go away, but she said it did bring her peace and closer to God.

As for me, I once more saw Christ working through my child and again was in awe. I got to experience firsthand through Cole and Doreen the blessing that is received when you truly trust in God and follow what he is asking you to do. This experience has made me become excited to listen for God's instructions and guidance in my life.

After that, we who are still alive and are left will be caught up together with them in the clouds to meet the Lord in the air. And so we will be with the Lord forever.

1 Thessalonians 4:17

Test of Faith

In August of 2002, Clay was out puddle-jumping with his aunt Laura. As he jumped over one particular puddle, Auntie Laura helped him over it by taking his hand and lifting him up. Unfortunately, his thumb got pulled out of place. We took him to the ER, where they were unsuccessful at pushing the thumb back into place. We had to come back the next day so they could put it back in by surgery. Imagine having to be put under anesthesia to push a thumb back into place! Leave it up to one of the Roberts boys to find a unique way into the surgery room.

Although it all seemed so unbelievable, I could not help but notice the fear Clay had going into that surgery room. Was it because he saw all that Cole had gone through, or was it a normal little boy's reaction to the unknown? I do know Clay's reaction made me realize that it does not matter how large or small a trial might be. What matters is how it is affecting the ones in it. One thing I knew I could count on was that God had gotten us through so many surgeries already that he would get us through this one also.

That was not the end of our August fun. Right after his thumb had healed, Clay and Cole were wrestling in the basement, and Clay broke his wrist! He was thrilled with his new cast because he thought it made him look tough. *Look tough?* With all that these boys had gone through so far in their short lives, Clay certainly did not need a cast to prove his strength. One moment I was looking at him in a cast, and the next minute I was filled with joy as I watched Clay interact with his friends at his fifth birthday party. He looked so small with his cast on yet so grown up blowing his candles out. My baby was growing up right before my eyes. I asked God at that moment to help me be the best mom I could for the boys, to have great strength in everything that comes our way in life to show them Christ.

Then, believe it or not, it was my turn to play patient. I was with the boys at

Wal-Mart when I felt a sudden and intense pain in my back. It felt like someone had stabbed me, so much so that I actually turned around and half expected to see someone with a knife. Immediately, we left Wal-Mart and drove to the nearest clinic. I can't for the life of me explain how I was able to drive with this sharp pain, but somehow I did. Once there, I called Mike's mom and dad to come get the boys for me. I was in too much pain to look after them, even in the waiting room.

I have always had to deal with cysts on my ovaries and had had surgeries on them in the past. In this case, the pain was caused by a cyst bursting open. I was rushed into emergency surgery.

While still recovering from that surgery, my tooth began to give me some trouble. I needed to get rid of the aching tooth and had to have a root canal. When that procedure was over, the dentist packed the space where my tooth had been extracted. But something was wrong. I was still in pain. In fact, the pain got worse. It was so excruciating I was throwing up and rapidly losing weight. *God, help me please. I cannot be sick; I have two boys to take care of.* I felt abandoned by him yet again. The fear that I could not take care of my boys was overwhelming to me. I spent the hours in bed praying for the miracle of healing.

Finally, after some time had passed, I went to a facial surgeon who X-rayed my face and found that when the dentist took out my tooth he had taken out too much of the bone behind it and put a hole in my sinuses. When the dentist put in the packing, it was pushed up into my sinuses, which caused the intense pain. The facial surgeon had to go in and repair the damage.

I was still getting sick from problems I was having with the cysts on my ovaries. It was decided that it was time for the hysterectomy I knew I needed. The surgery went well, but I was extremely nervous. Recovery from a hysterectomy is a long and painful process, so I prayed that nothing major would happen to the boys while I was recovering. I really did not know how I would be able to take care of anyone. My limitations were tested, however, when just three weeks after my surgery Cole started along another path of overcoming tragedy, and I had to find the strength to walk with him. My prayers turned to pleads for strength, faith, and courage. Still feeling like I was alone going from one medical problem to another, I asked myself, *Can God hear me? Maybe I am praying the wrong way.*

It was Labor Day weekend, and we were headed to Mike's parents' cabin on Otter Tail Lake in Minnesota. I couldn't tell you who was more excited, the boys or Mike. It was so refreshing to actually see everyone smiling and feeling somewhat better. I said a small prayer of thanks to God for our safe trip and the opportunity to have a nice weekend together. It was already early evening by the time we got there, and the boys could only think about getting into the water. Grandma Mary volunteered to take them down to the water, even though it was already getting a little dark and chilly. Cole, in his excitement, began to run as he reached the dock and tripped over a hole in the wood. He fell flat onto his stomach, but this did not slow him down. He was in the water within minutes and swam until we called him out.

As the boys were getting ready for bed, Cole told us he was getting a stomachache. I sat with him through the night, but his stomachache was not going away. My thoughts went back to the past few months. Cole had been battling what I thought was a stomach flu since July. He would be really sick and very tired. Then he would be fine for about a week before it would start all over again. This time, I thought that his pain was probably due to all the lake water he had accidentally drunk while swimming.

We must remember that Cole had had major reflux surgery to keep him from throwing up. In situations where most people would throw up, Cole had to wait for his system to re-route what needed to be eliminated into diarrhea. I was very familiar with Cole and the way his body worked, so I became anxious when time passed and he still did not show any signs of diarrhea. I was impatient because I knew that if he would only go to the bathroom he would feel better.

The nearest town was thirty minutes away, but Grandpa Herb wanted to go in search of some medication that would quicken the process. While he was gone, Cole said he felt the need to go to the bathroom. *Finally,* I thought, feeling bad that Grandpa Herb had apparently left for no reason. It was 3:30 a.m. when I led Cole to the bathroom. When Cole was done going to the bathroom, my relief quickly turned into horror as I saw the toilet was filled with blood. I yelled for Mike and his mom, as we all looked at each other with complete terror. We rushed to the car as fast as we could. The noise we made in that small lake community woke the others up. The relatives from our cabin and the cabin across the road came to our aid. They would watch Clay and let Grandpa Herb know what was going on. We raced to that town thirty minutes away and drove straight to the ER.

During this time of the unknown, I could only think that perhaps Cole had a very bad case of the flu. I think at that point God was keeping my thoughts away from all the terrible things that passing blood can mean because he wanted me to keep my head clear. Simple, non-threatening answers to Cole's loss of blood continued to entertain my thinking until the doctor came in with an X-ray he had taken of Cole. As he placed the X-ray up onto the light, my heart flipped. I saw it right away. I had seen it before, only this time it was much bigger. The cancerous tumor, Wilms, was back.

At that moment I could not hear, I could not think, I could not breathe. I had to get out of that room. I got up to leave, and the doctor turned to Mike and said, "You go help that mom right now!" Mike found me and just held me. He talked about pulling together so we could get Cole back home as fast as we could. This calmed me down enough to be able to call back to the relatives at the cabin. We asked those who waited for us to pack our things so that when we got there we could just go.

Cole was getting sicker and sicker. He was in a lot of pain, so we wanted to get to Bismarck as soon as possible. The doctor called the emergency room in our town to let them know what he had found. We called Grandpa Herb and let him know what was going on, and then we called the police to let them know we would be speeding from Minnesota to North Dakota and to not stop us.

It was a long and scary ride. So much went through my mind, and I honestly could not pray anymore. I just kept repeating over and over that same old chant, "God, why?" and "Please help."

Finally we pulled into the ER and waited anxiously as the doctor examined Cole. I almost fell over when he told us to go home and bring Cole back on Monday when he would be able to be looked at by a specialist. So we took him home. What choice did we have? As I sat there watching my son getting steadily worse, my anger grew. I could only take two hours of watching Cole suffer. We took him back to the hospital, and this time we said that we would not leave until a doctor came to see him. *None were coming!*

Out of desperation, I called Cole's pediatrician at her home. Despite the early morning call from a frantic mom, she was very sympathetic. She phoned the on call doctor, who then came in to look at Cole. Then she called the Mayo Clinic, a hospital in Rochester, Minnesota, that specializes in cancer patients, and soon an ambulance arrived to take Cole there.

I felt helpless as they placed Cole into the back of the ambulance. He was in pain, and he was gagging and dry heaving. There was nothing the doctors could give him to relieve him of this awful nightmare. Mike rode with Cole in the ambulance, and his parents, Clay, and I followed behind in the car. It was another long night, and I was tired and scared. One blessing I had that kept me going was when I would look in my rearview mirror and see Clay laying in the backseat trying to sleep. He looked just like an angel. I felt in my heart that was

God telling me to keep going; he was in control and would get us there safe.

We stopped a few times on the outskirts of large cities for the paramedics to check on Cole and make sure he was stable enough to go on. When they got the okay, we were off again. During one of these stops, which I personally thought were a waste of time, they called in to see if they could give Cole anything for the severe pain he was in. Only Benadryl was allowed to try to calm him down. One great blessing was that we knew a friend who was a paramedic, and she agreed to do the transport with us. This gave us great comfort to know Cole was in good hands. I also looked at it as one more little gift from God saying, "I am with you always."

We arrived in Rochester, and things seemed to go so fast, and yet at the same time, it was all moving in slow motion. We met with a whirlwind of doctors, one after another. They placed a tube in Cole's nose that went down to his stomach. This tube had to stay in for a few days before they could do any type of surgery. Its purpose was to remove all the food and such out of his system because his body had shut down and was not able to do it on its own. As I looked at Cole with all the tubes in, I asked God to give me a sign that all would be okay, but either I did not get one or I could not see through all the pain to find it.

During all this, one of the nurses found out I had a hysterectomy three weeks earlier. She looked at me in surprise then yelled out to the other nurses, "Get a cot in here; this mother is three weeks post op!" A cot was brought in, and I was ordered to use it. I was told I should have never been carrying my son. How could

I not? How can you keep a mother who just found out her boy had cancer from holding and serving him?

The days spent waiting for Cole to be stable enough for surgery were a mini roller coaster inside of the giant coaster we were already on. Events and emotions were constantly rising, falling, and spinning. One day, I would be in the chapel lighting a candle for Cole and feeling such a peace of God's presence, and the next day I felt I was going to lose my mind completely.

At last Cole was stable enough to remove the kidney and the tumor. There were no complications during the surgery, and all went well. We were informed that the cancer was in stage one, phase one. Praise God! When getting this news, I knew right away that was the sign I was praying for, the sign that all was going to be okay.

After praising God, I asked him to forgive me for my times of doubt and if he would help me stay strong and focused on him during the days to come, good or bad. I heard him in my heart that day say, "I am here and will never leave." I prayed that I would always remember those words.

Be joyful in hope, patient in affliction, and faithful in prayer.

Romans 12:12

O Lord, the God who saves me, day and night I cry out before you. May my prayer come before you; turn your ear to my cry.

Psalm 88:1–2

The Dreaded Chemo

Time was spent in the hospital getting Cole strong once more, and during this time we met a lot of very nice people and even made a friend or two. I will never forget the day I looked down the hall, and there was Clay riding on the lap of another boy who did not have legs. They were having a great time cruising through the halls of the hospital. With all that the boys were experiencing, God was teaching them to not be afraid of others who have disabilities. Yet another blessing in disguise was being poured out over us.

We took Cole home in a van that had a mattress placed in the back so he could lie down. This was important because he had been cut from side to side during the surgery and we did not want the stitches to tear open.

The next step in this journey was chemotherapy. I can honestly say I was never so scared in my life—scared of the unknown, scared what was going to happen to Cole, just plain scared and in disbelief that my son was going to have to have chemo. Cole would get the treatments every Friday for ten months. During this time, I was extremely concerned about Cole's environment being germ free because he would not have an immune system to fight with. This, for me, was a very overwhelming thought. He had to have a port surgically placed into his chest. A port is a device that a needle can be put into so the nurses would not have to find a blood vein every week. The whole chemotherapy procedure would take two hours from start to finish.

As the Fridays piled up behind us, we began to dread the end of every week. I am amazed as I think about all the times I complained about these awful visits to Mike or even just to myself, and yet I never heard one complaint from Cole. Oh, he cried, felt sick to his stomach, and was tired of the whole ordeal, but he never voiced any "poor me" thoughts. He never had fits of anger, nor did he verbalize how he felt in a negative way. I wished I could have been half as strong as he was.

One of my hardest days was when Cole was eating what little he could. He stopped and said, "Mommy, I think I got a hair in my mouth." Horrified, I stared at the first chunk of hair that had fallen out from the chemo. From that moment on I looked at Cole differently. No longer was he Cole, my son who has cancer and this is what we do. Now he was Cole, my son who has cancer and I might lose him. I felt every pain, every stomachache, every tear, and every fear deep in my heart as it was breaking. *Where is God?*

Like so many times before, one minute I could feel him, and the next I could not. The question of, "Why God? Why?" was followed by, "Hasn't Cole been through enough? He has been taken from school, put through surgery after surgery, robbed of sight, and now stripped of his hair, which left him with the look of chemo, and to me that was the look of death. How can I keep my faith?" I did not know how; I just knew I had to. Everything we were going through was so hard, but I knew it would be unbearable to do it without him.

For three days we dealt with hair falling out. Sometimes it fell out in large clumps, sometimes smaller ones. It came to the point where Cole asked me to shave his head. We stood in the shower, razor in hand. Cole was excited about this new adventure of having a bald scalp; after all, his dad was bald as well. This excitement faded as the reality of the situation hit Cole. He began to cry as I shaved off what was left of his hair. I tried to speak soothing, encouraging words into his ear as I worked. When it was over, I held him, and we cried on the bathroom floor together. After that, Cole never said any more about his hair and the great pain of losing it that day.

The more Fridays that went by, the sicker Cole became. He lost a lot of weight and was very thin. Every week it was the same nightmare. Fridays, of course, were chemo days. Saturdays Cole was very tired and sick. Sundays were the same as Saturdays. Mondays he would feel a little better. Tuesdays were his worst days for being sick. Wednesdays were like Mondays. Thursdays Cole would feel better but could not enjoy it because he knew the next day it would start all over again.

A bright spot on those terrible chemo Fridays was that my dad would take off of work, come to the hospital, and give Cole wheelchair rides, complete with wheelies, up and down the hallway; he would also read to Cole to help pass the time and fear. That made chemo much easier to deal with for Cole and for me. It was also comforting to Mike, knowing that a man was there looking out for Cole and giving me support in his stead. Mike was unable to take off those Fridays because he had to save all his vacation days for emergency runs out of town, which always seemed to pop up.

One thing I regret during that time of chemo was being talked into having tutors come over once a week to do schoolwork. I realize now that the work was not as important as feeling well and resting. Cole missed seventy-two days of his first grade year. He did, however, with a lot of hard work and determination, catch up with his class, so he did not need to repeat that grade.

The days, weeks, and months that Cole suffered through chemo were a hard mountain to climb. I watched as Cole's life was being slowly pumped out with every push of the chemo drug into his veins. I watched as my son began to show all the signs of someone with cancer. His body was thin and his face pale with dark circles around his eyes. I imagined this must have been what walking death looked like. A mom's job is to kiss the pain and hurt and make them go away, but there was no Band-Aid big enough to heal this. I didn't know what to do or even how to handle being scared.

You would think that with all the concerns I had with Cole I wouldn't be concerned with how others saw me or what they thought about how I was handling things. Quite the opposite was true. I worried about how I was expected to feel and act. I tried to perform how others thought I should perform and feel how they thought I should be feeling, from what I should or should not cry about to whether I was crying too much or not enough. I struggled with how I spent the little free time I had. Did I spend enough of it on my own to get recharged, or was that being selfish? I even worried about my appearance. I did not want to look too good, and I did not want to look like I was not able to take care of myself either. I spent too much time trying to be who I believed people wanted me to be instead of allowing myself to focus on how I truly felt and acting on that. I regret that I looked to others for cues on what to say and do instead of looking to God as my guide.

At this time in my life, I honestly think that I still

held some anger and hurt toward God. Deep down I wanted to live my life for him but truly was not strong enough to allow myself to surrender the path that was put before me and trust him. When you hold anger toward someone, the last thing you want to do is talk to them, let alone ask them for advice. This is where I was with God. I could pray for things, but I could not receive the things he was giving to me. If only I could have been at the place in my life I am today. Would it have made it any easier? I do not know. I do know, though, that I would have had more peace.

I also worried about Clay. He was just as scared as the rest of us about Cole, and yet I never seemed to have enough time to spend just being his mom. I wished I could have torn myself in two so I could give Cole my undivided attention in his time of need and Clay the attention every little boy deserves from his mother. Cancer had placed Clay on the backburner of our lives and stolen family fun time away from him as well as the rest of us. I asked God to keep his hand on Clay and let him know that I loved him so very much.

Helpless, the only thing I could do was pray. I prayed so much it became more like a mantra, the same thing every day and every hour. This prayer, this chant, molded itself into everything I did and thought until it became who I was. God is good, and even in the most trying of times, he brings us happy memories. It was during this time that we were the recipients of much needed love and encouragement from our church. We were constantly reminded that we were being held up in prayer by fellow parishioners. Many visited and inquired about how we were doing. It was their concern and thoughtfulness that kept God alive for me as I struggled to understand this journey.

Even outside of the church, we were shown a great

deal of compassion, and the desire to help us was made known by many in the community. It is pretty common that chemo patients find they are only able to tolerate certain foods while undergoing treatment. Cole was no exception, and his miracle food was doughnuts. It was amazing how many people had heard this and brought us Krispy Kremes all the way from Fargo. Even strangers would drop by to hand Cole these prized delicacies. In all, we received thirty dozen doughnuts, and each one looked like pure gold to me because as he ate each doughnut I knew he was getting *something* in his stomach to keep his body going.

I will also hold dear to my heart the time spent with Cole in the hammock or on the couch reading, as well as the many wagon rides we took together. I loved this time that we were able to spend together. Of course, I would have preferred doing these things without Cole being so sick, but if I am honest, I don't think I would have taken the time if he was a normal healthy child.

The cords of death entangled me; the torrents of destruction overwhelmed me. The cords of the grave coiled around me; the snares of death confronted me. In my distress I called to the Lord; I cried to my God for help. From his temple he heard my voice; my cry came before him, into his ears.

Psalm 18:4–6

Code Blue

In October, Cole took a turn for the worse. He was even more pale and weak than usual. He ended up in the hospital and was given fluids for several days. He did not have to go in for chemo that week so his body would have a chance to build itself back up. As soon as he felt strong enough, he started chemo once again, which was not easy for me. I couldn't help but wonder if the horrific chemo drug would kill him, even if it was meant to save his life. The cancer had been taken out with the kidney; was all this torment really necessary?

It seemed after that time spent in the hospital Cole continued to go downhill. He was getting sicker and sicker and had to go back to the hospital several times for more fluids. Cole's doctor had wanted him to start seeing a psychiatrist, because many people who endure chemo treatments become depressed. We took his advice and went to a psychiatrist who immediately placed Cole on medication. In fact, at one time, he was taking seven to ten different drugs.

In December, Cole ended up in the hospital again, where he started having grand mal seizures. These seizures were so intense that sometimes it would take three of us to hold him down in bed. This would happen pretty much non-stop, from right after he was given his medication at 5:00 p.m. until well into the night. I could not believe this was happening. What more was one child supposed to endure? I felt so helpless because I did not know how to stop this. I did, however, for the first time in a long time, feel no anger toward God, and even though so much was happening, I felt a peace. Not peace with what Cole was going through but a much deeper peace—it was the presence of God.

Many people from the church came and prayed for him constantly. At one point, some of them went into the lobby to pray fervently for Cole because it looked almost like he had a demon-like spirit oppressing him. This helped so much, just to know that people cared enough about us to spend their time praying out loud in a hospital lobby for my son. This was a true testimony to me of God's love and their faithfulness in him.

The situation kept getting worse. We tried calling the doctor over and over, but she would not come in because it happened to be a weekend. We called her at home, and the nurses did as well. She still would not come in to see Cole and instead said that it was probably anxiety and told the nurses to up his medication. When this still did not seem to work, she called Cole's psychiatrist, who came in only to give him even more medication.

Cole began losing control of his bodily functions. He could not control his bladder or bowels, could not walk on his own, and could not talk. He would spit, and foam would come out of his mouth. At this point I was numb; I honestly cannot tell you what I was feeling. I reached a point of not knowing what I was feeling because it was so intense. I can only explain it like this: you will hear about people who are going through a lot of trauma becoming numb to it or blocking out what is happening to them. This is what I was doing and not even realizing it.

After two nights of this, we threatened that if Cole's doctor did not come in immediately we would take him somewhere else. Reluctantly she arrived, and when she saw the condition Cole was in, she started taking the situation more seriously; in fact, she began to panic. She gave Cole seizure medication and was constantly on the phone to the Mayo Clinic. She did all this without once looking Mike or me in the eye.

Cole's psychiatrist showed up unexpectedly but refused to come into Cole's room. Instead he called us out into the hallway where he dropped a bombshell on us. They had been overdosing Cole! He had errantly prescribed Cole an adult dosage of medication. That medication had been doubled because a nurse had forgotten to write down that he was already taking this drug. Also, the pharmacy did not catch that they were dispensing too much of this drug and did not take into consideration the mixture of all the other medications Cole was taking. All that and the fact that Cole had lost so much weight due to chemotherapy made the overdoses even more devastating.

I was so mad, mad at the fact that my son was suffering because of someone else's mistake. If only things could have been different, if only someone would have caught this mistake before he suffered. I tried telling myself, *They are only human; we all make mistakes.* This did not work; I was angry and did not know how to stop being angry.

Cole was air ambulanced immediately to the Mayo Clinic. I flew with Cole while Mike, his parents, and Clay all drove down together. I hated being separated from Mike again, especially when I needed him so much. The flight nurses continually worked on Cole in the jet ambulance trying to control the seizures. At one point they said, "We have a code blue in progress." They got the paddles ready as they rapidly gave him medication to bring his heart rate back up. The medication worked, and the paddles were put away.

When we landed, they took Cole from my sight, and I was not allowed to stay with him. Once again, I found myself alone waiting. I was in a room with no phone and no way to talk to Mike or anybody else. The desire to see and be with Cole was stronger than I had ever felt before, maybe because I had never been so close to losing him. I had time to reflect in that room on what just happened. How close was I to watching my son die right before my eyes? Even as they worked so hard in another room, would everything turn out *okay?* Or were we too late? I did not have Mike there to comfort me with words of hope. Clay was not there to blissfully distract me from my own thoughts.
In my isolation, I felt the powerful need to have my family together. It seemed I was in that room for a long time, but in reality, I suppose it was only about forty-five minutes. Then I was led into a big ICU room with a little crib-like bed, surrounded by wires, buttons, nurses, and doctors. They had already done a brain scan, and they said his little brain looked like the brain of an adult male drug user that had just overdosed.

Cole was resting, so I just held his hand as tears streamed down my face. The doctors were asking so many questions, and I could not believe how angry they were about all of the medications Cole had been given. At one point I felt like they were mad at me for letting it happen. After all of the questions and a few more tests, Cole and I were alone. I thanked God for letting me stay with him and prayed that his brain would not be damaged from the many days of seizures it had endured.

Cole was taken off all the medications that were prescribed to him and was given instead a medicine that would counteract the side effects of the earlier medications, and they pushed fluids through his system at a high speed to get the bad medicine out. In less than twenty-four hours, Cole was talking, smiling, and even laughing. He was his old self once again, but he was extremely tired. We were in that hospital for a few more days before we were able to go home.

Mike and I wanted to end Cole's chemotherapy right then and there. The chemo included a drug called Vincristine, which, because the doctors did not adjust the dosage after Cole had lost a lot of his weight, was one of the causes of his seizures. Unfortunately, we were persuaded into continuing on with the chemo treatments and controlling the seizures with seizure medication. Cole would start on chemo again, but this time with only half the dosage of his regular treatments.

When Cole began to have seizures once more, we stopped chemotherapy completely; however, the effects of chemotherapy lingered. Cole began to lose feeling in his fingers. We were furious that we were not told this would be a side effect of the chemo. If Cole couldn't feel with his fingers, he couldn't read!

He continued to have small seizures for two years. He had to be on seizure medication, which had its own set of side effects, for three years. His legs ached, and he did not have reflexes in them for almost one year after stopping the chemo. This made it hard for him to balance. The chemo also had caused his veins to collapse easily, so anytime he needed blood drawn, it would take several pokes to find a good vein. This also made it difficult to have any IVs put in. The veins would hold up for a little while but would eventually fall. His bones became very weak as well; he had broken or fractured his arm three times. I hated how it affected his life; he had no energy and would get sick if he overdid it or got the slightest bit worn down. This would happen so easily. A normal get-together with friends could make him sick for a few days after. To this day he has to be careful not to get run down.

It took the better part of four years before we were able to see all the side effects of Cole's chemotherapy completely disappear. These side effects were getting feeling back into his fingers, which was a blessing so he could continue to read Braille, reflexes back into his legs, which helped with balance, and his bones did not break so easily anymore. On the upside, Cole's hair came back dark, curly, and thick. Ah, the wonderful little rainbows God gives us after the flood.

In September of 2003, we went back to Otter Tail Lake. We had gone full circle. It had been one year since an angel had pushed Cole on that pier and saved his life. We wanted to say thank you. Without that push, the tumor would have not gotten agitated, and we would not have found it in time to save Cole's life. Also, we wanted to bring closure to the entire journey. We did this by facing the lake together as a family and then spitting into it. People laugh when we tell them we did this, but really, it was all quite freeing. It was difficult when all the horrible memories came flooding back as we stood by the lake, but we dealt with it and it brought us closer together.

Standing there looking at the lake beside my family, I reflected on how water was used for so much good in the Bible, from baptism to protection. That day so long ago Cole's life was saved from the fall he took at the lake on the water's edge, and now with him alive and standing beside me, the water would give us memories of hope and the triumph over cancer. God is good and faithful.

Then we made more memories there. We had a great time, and it was those happy memories of Otter Tail Lake that we took home with us this time.

We do not want you to be uninformed, brothers, about the hardships we suffered in the province of Asia. We were under great pressure, far beyond our ability to endure, so that we despaired even of life. Indeed, in our hearts we felt the sentence of death. But this happened that we might not rely on ourselves but on God, who raises the dead. He has delivered us from such a deadly peril, and he will deliver us. On him we have set our hope that he will continue to deliver us, as you help us by your prayers. Then many will give thanks on our behalf for the gracious favor granted us in answer to the prayers of many.

2 Corinthians 1:8–11

Open Heart Surgery

Two things Cole had always wanted to do were go to Disney World and to swim with the dolphins. He was selected to have his wish granted from the Make-a-Wish Foundation, and in January 2004, he chose to go to Disney World.

It was such a wonderful gift. We were in the Magic Kingdom, and magical it was. We were treated like royalty. Everything was planned for us to make every minute of the trip special. It was arranged so that we did not have to stand in the long lines at the theme parks, the fridge in the little cottage we stayed in was stocked with the boys' favorite foods, and every night when we would get back from all our sightseeing, there would be a little gift on the table for both Clay and Cole. The Mayor Bunny would come tuck them into bed at night. I loved how they made Clay feel special right along with his brother. I was so thankful that they understood how scary it can be for a sibling to watch his brother go through all Cole was going through.

We met so many of the Disney characters and Universal Studio characters from Shrek to Mickey Mouse himself! I was touched to see that every one of the characters would get down on Cole's level so he could feel every inch of their costumes, right there in the middle of the busy streets. I will never forget how free we felt, almost like we were just another normal family. I did not want to leave. I wanted to live in the village forever, not because of how we were treated, but because for those few days it was like Cole could see, and sickness had no way of entering our lives or our thoughts. There were so many people who made this amazing trip a reality for us: the Make-a-Wish Foundation; the Give Kids the World organization; and Mike's coworkers, who had collected money to pay for Cole to swim with the dolphins on his ninth birthday.

Most of 2004 was fairly uneventful. Cole had a lot of sinus problems, which finally ended in sinus surgery, with the possibility of more sinus surgeries down the road. We had small, normal kid sicknesses, which were looked at as a blessing because it made us feel normal to have just a typical cold. As 2004 was coming to an end, however, we were faced once again with another journey. This time it was Clay's mountain to climb.

In December of that year, Clay, who was seven, had been complaining that his throat was hurting him. After he had told us this, I did notice he was rather pale and seemed to be getting tired easily. I was not too concerned, though. I thought it might be due to his asthma. I took him in to see the doctor, thinking his sore throat could have been strep throat. The test for strep came back negative, so we thought it was probably just a virus.

Days went by and Clay was getting worse. I took him to the clinic two more times that week, and two more times we were sent home with no knowledge of what could be causing his sore throat. Clay could hardly eat because of the pain, and by Friday, he was pretty weak. On Saturday, Clay begged me to take him to the doctor one more time. On the car ride over, I felt something was wrong in the pit of my stomach. I began to argue with it in my head. *It is just a virus,* I told that nagging feeling. *This is a waste of time.*

At the ER, the doctor asked questions concerning what might be the cause of this pain. We told him that on Thursday Clay had taken a NyQuil pill and it had gotten caught in his throat. Clay was able to get it down, but the doctor said this could have scratched or even burned Clay's esophagus. He decided to do an upper GI. Clay had to drink a thick, white liquid, and the doctor watched as it went down using an X-ray type of machine. Even though Clay was scared and in pain, he drank all the liquid like a trooper.

Clay and I went back to his ER room while the doctor reviewed the results of the GI. Clay was blissfully watching television, but I was starting to get uneasy. I had been in the ER enough times to know that when it takes as long as it was taking, something is wrong. I could no longer just sit, so I quickly ran to the door and stuck my head out. I was nervous and hoped to see the doctor in the halls.

At last the doctor came into the room and sat down. He told Clay that the good news was nothing was stuck in his throat. There was, however, something pushing on his throat from the outside. We needed to do a CT scan to see what it was. Knowing that Clay had been feeling sick, the doctor was hopeful it was only an enlarged lymph node.

A wave of nausea came over me, and I ran out of the room and into the bathroom, where I instantly threw up. As I was washing up, I looked into the mirror, trying to get a grip on myself for Clay's sake. "Please, God," I prayed. "Not cancer. Not my healthy son."

The wait for the results of the CT scan was another long one. This was again to me an indication that something was seriously wrong.

When the doctor finally came in to talk to us, he

told us he had to call in a heart specialist to consult with. The CT scan showed that nothing was actually pushing on the esophagus, but rather the main aorta of Clay's heart was wrapped around it. This is a congenital condition called a vascular ring, and so the journey began.

Clay was put in the hospital because his oxygen level was really low and it needed to go back up before he could be sent to the Children's Hospital in Minnesota. The doctor wanted to send Clay there in an ambulance, but we had been down that road before and didn't want to do that again. It took a lot of convincing, but he finally agreed to let us take Clay to the hospital ourselves.

Mike, Clay, and I took off for Minnesota, and Cole stayed back with my parents. How strange it felt for the roles of the boys to be switched. When we arrived at the hospital, we went straight into the emergency room. We were very tired and very scared. It seemed like we sat and waited for hours. I was anxious to get the tests started so we could get answers to our many questions. Clay was given an EKG of his heart, an upper GI, and a CAT scan, among other tests, before he was placed in his own room.

The next day was Clay's surgery. We pulled him around in a little wagon in the hallways until it was his turn to go in. The whole time, Clay was shaking with fright; even his little teeth were rattling. One of the nurses noticed this and brought the doctor out to give Clay some medication to calm him down. This helped so very much, and he was able to rest with no fear. I remember looking at him in the wagon. It took me back straight to the time when I would push him in the stroller. So loving and precious, the face of a child.

When the time came to let him go into surgery, I could not stop crying. I knew it was going to be a long surgery and an unpleasant recovery. I was thankful for the medication that had calmed Clay down because it kept him from being aware of my sobs as they took him away. All of a sudden, it was just Mike and me in a crowded waiting room. We had been in a lot of waiting rooms, but this one was the worst we had ever seen. It was very small and set up in such a way that you couldn't really walk around. We were stuck in a room that didn't even have magazines to browse through.

I began to think of all the times we waited in a variety of rooms for surgeries to be over, and most of those times we had a brother and grandparents waiting with us. I felt that it was unfair to Clay that the only bodies in this room waiting to see him were that of Mike and me.

Time seemed to crawl, and it felt like we were in that waiting room for days. I did not know it while we were sitting in that cramped little room, but those hours spent waiting, just Mike and me, were quite a blessing. The two of us were able to help each other get through this latest challenge by knowing when to talk and when to just hold each other. Even though we both grieve and handle stress in totally different ways. Finally we were at a place in our lives that we could talk about our feelings and know when each other was not ready to talk but just needed to be held. Was this just because we were older? No, this was because we had started talking more and praying more together. Our faith was growing stronger not only as individuals but together as a couple. We were learning to work together and step out of our comfort zones to trust in each other and together trust in God.

When Clay's surgery was over and we were able to go to him, nothing or nobody could have prepared me for what I saw. Clay was hooked up to a large, very loud, very scary-looking respirator machine. He was so very tiny, and there were tubes and cords everywhere. If they told me Clay would be on this machine, I had completely forgotten. A nurse interrupted my panicked gaze and began listing many instructions for Mike and me to follow: keep him calm, tell him to not talk, and tell him to not move. I was thinking, *Okay, and how am I supposed to do that?*

When Clay's eyes began to open, we started right away to tell him to not try to talk. We told him to not fight the machine that was breathing for him. We did our best to explain everything we could to him. Clay was extremely brave and listened very well. He did not fight at all, even though, by the tears running down his face, he was very scared.

We were told that he might need the respirator for fifteen to twenty hours after the surgery, and if he did well, they would slowly turn the machine down every hour. By the grace of God, Clay only had the respirator on for four to five hours. Every so often, during that time, a tear would fall from his little eyes. I asked him if he was in any pain, but he would shake his head no. I just kept praying, "Please, God, do not let him have any pain."

When they took his breathing tube out, he did exactly what they told him to do, and it came out fast. He did not have much pain and was very alert and talking. He asked a lot of questions but did not want to laugh because it was very painful to do so.

Years later, I would find out that he was more scared being on that machine than we had ever imagined. The terror of waking up to find himself connected to that monster of a respirator was so traumatic because he could not speak to ask the questions he had. Like, would the tube hurt when they pulled it out? And would he never be able to talk again? I felt so bad that I did not think of the questions that were haunting his little mind. The relief of being off that machine was so great for him, as well as for us, that we underestimated the fear Clay had experienced. For us it was another little prayer answered. I truly believe God knew we would need things to go smoothly because with all we had been through with the surprise of the respirator and the fear Clay was experiencing, our strong faith and trust in him could start to diminish.

It was painful for Clay to walk, but his doctors wanted him to. When it was time for Clay to go to the bathroom, he was told that he needed to walk to it. He was scared, so Mike helped him out. Mike stood behind him and scooped him up in such a way that Clay was sitting in his hands. Then Mike let Clay's feet touch the floor ever so slightly so it looked like he was walking. We did not get away with that for very long. The next day, he was told to walk the length of the ICU room. Clay was still scared, so Mike told him that if he walked the length of the room, he would buy him an Xbox. Well, Clay became one determined little boy. He dug deep and walked through all of the pain. To this day, Clay loves to tell people the story of how he got his Xbox, and I love to tell how God helped him walk.

Once back home, I was still very anxious. I had an unrelenting fear that Clay's heart would stop. Even though the doctors assured me he was now all better, I could not help but to worry that Clay's procedure would come undone. I did not want him to wrestle, run, walk, or even talk for fear of something happening to him again.

I became encouraged as I saw him grow and be more active every day. His energy came back, as well as the color in his face. Despite my fears and worries, Clay healed amazingly fast. In fact, we soon discovered that his strength returned faster than anyone expected. Clay and Mike had just come back from a follow-up doctor's appointment, where they were told that Clay was not to wrestle for two or three more weeks. The two of them stopped at the school to let the wrestling coach know the doctor's orders, and while Mike was still talking to the coach, he looked down the mats and saw Clay wrestling aggressively with one of his teammates without any signs of hesitation. Mike just watched in amazement and wonder at the strength he saw in his son. It was at that moment Mike knew with certainty Clay was going to be all right. I think the funny part of that story was the fear Mike had of telling me what had happened in that wrestling room.

Soon after that, he was wrestling again and doing very well. He made it to the state championships, where he lost in the freestyle match only by one. He won, however, in the Greco and Folk style matches, but more importantly, he won over the fears and anxiety of heart surgery.

Sometimes as I look back on the whole thing, I am still amazed at how God created us. The doctors were able to open Clay up and work on his heart, and then in no time he was wrestling. I thank God for this miracle because to me even though Clay was not miraculously healed, I truly believe God gave us the miracle of healing through the doctor's hands.

The rest of the year 2005 was great. Clay was growing a lot and eating better. Then out of nowhere, the pain came back in 2006. Another upper GI was taken, and it was discovered that the area where the esophagus and trachea had been pinched together from the aorta being wrapped around them was weak. Because of this, Clay was having reflux problems. Also, because Clay had this condition since birth, he had learned to swallow differently than you or I do. As he swallowed, he would hold some food in his throat, allowing only a little to go down at a time so the pain would not be so bad. If we were to do this, we would gag on the food in our esophagus. Clay did not gag anymore but would actually hold his breath while he swallowed.

Clay was given high doses of Prevacid, an anti-reflux medicine, and started swallow therapy, which would last six months. He did not enjoy therapy, but we saw a great deal of improvement with his eating, and we were all thankful for that. However, not all of Clay's therapy was related to throat problems. The therapist also had him do reading and math. She felt that Clay's oxygen deprivation could have played a role in his struggles with schoolwork.

This same therapist also diagnosed Clay, my eight-year-old, of being too much of a mama's boy. I had to disagree with her. I felt that with everything Clay had gone through and watched his brother go through, his closeness to me was very natural. I needed a second opinion and took Clay to see a Christian counselor. It was her opinion that there is no such thing as a mama's boy unless you are in your thirties and still being spoon-fed. She believed that wanting to feel safe and being with his family were not signs of being a mama's boy.

When Clay stopped going to swallow therapy, his whole outlook had changed. He was back to his smiling self, was eating well, and was actually gaining weight. He still every now and again was fearful of what he ate, but he was given a clean bill of health and wouldn't need to be back to see the doctor for a whole year. At that time, he would have another cardiogram. If the cardiogram came out okay, then Clay would no longer need any more checkups for his heart.

This bit of information was encouraging, but it also shook me up a bit. I was under the impression that after a major heart surgery like what Clay had you would want to have regular checkups just to make sure everything was still working all right. I decided I needed to trust that everything would be all right. I rested in the fact that Clay was strong, healthy, and doing very well.

I also prayed that God would give me the insight when things were not right with the boys, not only medically but also emotionally. I never again want to miss the struggle Clay had emotionally with the swallow doctor. I asked Clay to forgive me for not catching it right away, or should I say not believing him when he would say that he did not like it or need it and that he was uncomfortable there. Like a true little man of God, he did not hesitate to give me forgiveness. I thank God every day for the strong role he has in my boy's life.

My health may fail and my spirit may grow weak, but God remains the strength of my heart; He is mine forever.

Psalm 73:26

The Storm

When Clay was still going through swallow therapy, Cole was beginning to show signs of distress. He was experiencing headaches, body aches, body sweats, and fatigue. We went through all the usual testing, MRI, CAT scan, and ultrasound. Cole, my dad, and I spent a week in Minnesota doing even more tests, everything from seizure tests to an advanced MRI. The doctors and nurses had him running in the hallways to tire out his body so they could witness the dizziness, stomachaches, sweating, and diarrhea that occurred.

It was another frustrating week of watching Cole suffer through tests and illness without the benefit of knowing why it was happening all while having our family separated yet again. After all that, the symptoms disappeared as quickly as they had come on.

As the year 2006 came to an end, I looked back at all the years that were behind us. They all seemed like a huge dream. I tried to pinpoint one specific year that was worse than all the others, with sickness, hospital visits, and surgeries, but I could not. In fact, they just all ran together endlessly. Now, as I write this, I do not look back to figure out which year was the worst, but rather I look for all the blessings we encountered from each of those years and every trial. It has been such a joy to see the boys grow through their life trials and experiences into independent young men filled with faith.

So much had happened in our lives that I felt we might need a way to sort it all out emotionally. We started to go to Clay's Christian counselor as a family on a regular basis. Through those sessions, we were able to discover a certain freedom from our pain and struggles. In this freedom I could see God's hand in everything that had happened to us. I wished I could have recognized it at the time, but maybe I had to come through it and grow to actually see it.

Our family structure began to make a change for the better. It was amazing. Our faith grew deeper both individually and together. We started to pray together more on a regular basis and not just the normal prayers before meals and bed but daily prayers for each other and family decisions. We all started to get more involved at church as individuals and also as a family unit. Our communication level increased; we started to communicate about everything, from our day, our thoughts, to what I feel was the most important, the way we handled conflicts. The peace and joy of becoming a family with deeper connections flowed over me.

The changes were so lovely and the harvest they were reaping so incredible that I feel truly blessed. Finally after so much heartache and "Why us, God?" I feel peace, trust, and a complete desire to surrender everything to him, for I know now it may not seem like it or it may be hard to see God in the storm, but he is there.

2007 started out very good. Clay, now nine, was doing better than ever. He was growing like a weed physically and emotionally and was becoming confident in who he was and who he wanted to be. School was going great for both of them. Both boys had wonderful teachers, and we as a family were closer than ever. Then, out of that dark place that always seems to linger so closely, illness attacked Cole once again.

His symptoms were severe, making his twelfth summer a very painful and unpleasant one. Mike and I were frightened at the thought of what could be causing these symptoms. Cole was continuously suffering from one thing or another. We started a journal in which we recorded all he was going through so we could keep our facts straight.

Summer symptoms: The following symptoms would occur on many but not all of the days of the following months.

May—Headaches, pale, tired all day, feeling pressure above his eyes, sweating excessively, dizzy, and stomachaches. On one occasion, Cole had his arm under his desk at school and it was rigid and shaking.

June—Pressure, pale, dizzy, headaches—some severe, pounding in the head, hot, very tired, diarrhea, lack of energy to do even the things he loved most such as swimming and playing with friends, would sweat excessively when doing minimal exercise.

July—Very moody, no ambition, easily agitated, very tired to the point that he felt he would fall down from exhaustion, lethargic—would sleep for excessive amounts of time and sometimes we were not able to wake him, diarrhea, got sick after a MRI, needed lots of rest after just a minimal amount of activity, loss of memory, arms held stiff with excessive shaking, very emotional, dizzy, mind feeling fuzzy, stomachaches, and pulsing pain.

—On one of these days, Cole was talking obsessively about a chair in a way that did not make any sense. Later, he did not remember this but was extremely dizzy.

Obviously, the summer was filled with difficulty. There was a big decline in Cole's desire to be with friends and do the things he loved. When he would engage in an activity, he would become very sick within an hour. This had been going on so long and so consistently that even Cole was getting frightened. He began to wonder if he would ever get better enough to play with his friends again.

Thankfully, August was much kinder to Cole. He experienced only a few headaches and was not as tired as he had been for most of the summer. He was able to play with friends a little bit more as well.

Although he was feeling better, we still went to the Children's Hospital in Minnesota to see if we could get answers to Cole's summer problems, and we took the journal with us. Once again, Cole faced a barrage of tests—MRI, CT, ultrasounds, seizure, blood, spinal fluid, urine, and sleep tests.

What they found was terrifying. Two spots were located on Cole's brain. They were both inoperable, so we were unable to take a biopsy to see if they were cancerous or not. The doctors could not even be positive that these spots were the cause of all of Cole's symptoms. So there we were, not knowing much and facing more questions than answers. We continued to do CT scans, but the medication they used was making Cole constantly sick and he asked us to stop.

Due to this request, we switched from CT testing to MRI scans, which revealed the spots had stopped growing, *praise God!* Just like that, after months of pain, frustration, doctor visits, tests, and prayers, the symptoms simply vanished. Similar to what had happened in 2006.

At first I was really irritated by the whole thing. Why go through all that only to have everything stop without doing anything or knowing anything? When I had time to catch my breath and really ponder what just happened, I realized the symptoms stopped as soon as the spots stopped growing. Perhaps the reason he was feeling better was because prayers had been answered. Even though this time was very scary and it was hard to see Cole go through all he did, there was a difference in all of us compared to past trials. We all surrendered every part of that journey to God and put it completely in his hands. Did this stop the worry, fear, or pain? No, but there was peace and fortitude that had never accompanied trial before.

We continued to pray for guidance as Cole was requesting to no longer have the spots scanned. He did not want to go through testing and hospital visits when, if in fact, there would be nothing the doctors could do even if the spots started to grow again. In the end we decided it was Cole's decision to make.

I know there are many who would not agree that Cole, at age twelve, should be allowed to make such a big decision; however, he is the one who had suffered through the many, many surgeries and tests. Yes, he was only twelve, but he was very smart and mature for that age. He had gone through so much already and understood his body more than anyone else could. Mike and I had watched as he went through all that he did, and we fully trusted that Cole, with God as his guide, was very capable of making that decision.

The rest of 2007 went really well. It is amazing how you can go through months in a storm of pain and uncertainty, and then all of a sudden everything is calm. Everything is going great, and you begin to get a feeling that your family might be becoming normal, whatever that may be.

Show me your ways, O Lord, teach me your paths; guide me in your truth and teach me, for you are God my Savior, and my hope is in you all day long.

Psalm 25:4–5

A Juggling Act

When 2008 rolled in, I felt as if I was performing a juggling act, trying to keep up the care of my two boys. Decisions I thought I would never have to make, like "Who do I take care of first?" needed to be made.

The juggling began when I noticed small amounts of blood on the floor of the bathroom and in the toilet. I asked if anyone had a bloody nose or if anyone had been bleeding for any reason. No one could tell me where the blood was coming from. I was not really concerned because the droplets were just here and there.

On January 20, Clay started getting awful stomachaches, a bad cough, and had pain above his eye. I was hoping and praying that this was just a cold or sinus infection.

January 21, I was taking a bath, and Cole came in to use the bathroom. That is when I saw the blood. I asked him if it hurt when he went to the bathroom. He said that it did, but not bad. On January 22, I took him in to see the local urologist. Cole's hypospadias that had been fixed when he was a baby had reopened. We scheduled surgery for the following week.

By January 23, the pain in Clay's eye was getting excruciating. We were trying anything and everything to get rid of that pain. After giving him medication, he would start to feel better, but it never took away the pain completely.

On January 24, Cole discovered a large lump on

his penis. It was very red and swollen with a small white center. We went in to see the doctor that same day, hoping this could get taken care of quickly, no matter what it was. I did not want to push back Cole's hypospadias surgery because the pain he was experiencing was getting worse, and I did not want his suffering to be prolonged.

Also on January 24, Clay called from school, wanting to come home. He was getting sick again and was in pain. Mike went to the school to be with him while I was with Cole at the clinic. I was so thankful Mike could take off to be with Clay.

Cole's doctor used a needle to open up the area where the lump was. He then proceeded to squeeze out a large white lump. Although this was a very painful process, Cole sat very still. When it was over, he felt very lightheaded and nauseous. His doctor assured us that those symptoms were only temporary and would go away. Sure enough, they did. Cole, feeling better, wanted to go back to school.

Clay wanted to finish his day at school as well. It was hard to leave both him and Cole, but I placed them both in God's hands as I left, knowing he would take good care of them. Once at home I got my Bible out and started to read.

I lift up my eyes to the hills—

Where does my help come from?

My help comes from the Lord,

The Maker of heaven and earth.

He will not let your foot slip—

He who watches over you will not slumber;

Indeed, he who watches over Israel

Will neither slumber nor sleep.

The Lord watches over you—

The Lord is your shade at your right hand;

The sun will not harm you by day,

Nor the moon by night.

The Lord will keep you from all harm—

he will watch over your life;

The Lord will watch over your coming and going

Both now and forevermore.

Psalm 121

This gave me the assurance of hope in God's protection. He watches over us and nothing diverts him.

I also read Psalm 123:

I lift up my eyes to you,

to you whose throne is in heaven.

As the eyes of slaves look to the hand of their master,

as the eyes of a maid look to the hand of her mistress.

so our eyes look to the Lord our God,

till he shows us his mercy.

Have mercy on us, O Lord, have mercy on us,

for we have endured much contempt.

We have endured much ridicule from the proud,

much contempt from the arrogant.

This Psalm confirmed in me the knowledge that when I lifted my eyes to God, looking for his mercy, he gave it to me because he loves us, and as Psalm 121 says, "He will never leave us."

When Cole went in for surgery to fix the hypospadias, he was extremely nervous. He shook uncontrollably until he was given some calming medication. The surgery went well, but Cole had to come home with a catheter. He had to keep that catheter in for eight days, and the first few days were really hard on him. By about day four, Cole had broken down in tears. He just had to cry and get out all of the frustrations of having to deal with pain, lack of sleep, missing school, and simply not being able to do anything.

Once Cole's catheter came out, he was in high spirits again and went back to school with no restrictions.

By February 9, Clay's eye was still giving him trouble, and his stomach never did get better. A doctor visit revealed that Clay had a bad sinus infection. It would take a while for the medications to fight off the infection, but what a relief to know the eye pain was due to sinuses and not the eye itself. These doctor visits, where the symptoms are easily diagnosed and treated, are indeed small miracles themselves. I was angered that it took so many doctor visits to figure this out, but glad; and thus, the juggling act was over, for now.

Trust in the Lord with all your heart and lean not on your own understanding.

Proverbs 3:5 NIV

The Tree

February 19, 2008, was a great day to go sledding. I took the boys and their friends to a nearby sledding hill. Cole, a teenager, did not want me out there with him and his friends. I stayed in the car but parked in a place where I was able to see the entire hill. At the bottom of the hill, there were some small trees, and my range of vision ended just beyond them.

Cole was doing great. I watched as he would sled down the hill, and upon reaching the bottom, he turned around and made his way back up to the top all by himself. At one point, I saw Cole go down the hill and get off his sled. Then I saw his friend go down and walk to Cole. Soon I did not see either of them and assumed they had gone into the tree area. Next thing I knew they were both walking to the car.

I was surprised they were finished sledding already, but then again, it was a pretty cold day. It wasn't until I noticed Cole holding his eye that I began to realize something was wrong. I ran to Cole and brought him back to the car. He told me that when he got to the bottom of the hill he had gotten turned around, and instead of running up the hill like he thought he was doing, he was running into the trees. In fact, he ran into a tree. The pain in his eye was so powerful after he hit the tree that he actually had passed out for a few seconds.

I looked into his eye but did not see a cut or any blood. Despite this incident, Cole did not feel like he had enough of sledding and wanted to go back out. I convinced him to rest for just a few minutes more. In that short time, he began to get a headache and wasn't feeling very good. Soon he was asking if we could leave. I gathered up the rest of the boys and took everyone home. When we got home, Cole let me look in his eye again. It was extremely red. I gave him some Advil and monitored it the rest of the night.

The next day, I took him to the eye doctor, where it was discovered that a small branch had gone right into Cole's eye. Apparently, with Cole thinking he was heading uphill with nothing in his way, he had his eyes wide open. Since he could not see the branch and was not expecting it, he did not have the reflex to close his eyes, and the branch went right in. Trauma to the eye like this causes so much pain that the blood pressure drops, and that is what made Cole pass out.

Cole was given eye drops to control the pain, but they did not work. We were told there was a chance his eye was so damaged that it might have to be removed. I struggled to not cry in front of Cole, but this was the last thing we wanted done. We had learned long ago that if scientists ever find a way to perform eye transplants, Cole would need his eye intact in order to have a transplant. In other words, as long as Cole had his eyes, there was a hope he might one day see again on this earth.

Immediately, I called everyone I could and asked for a bombardment of prayer.

Cole was in a lot of pain and was asking to just take out the eye so the pain would stop. All the growth I had accomplished in trusting God went by the wayside for a while. It finally took me getting completely down on my face before God to get back on track. It was so amazing; as soon as I surrendered all possible thoughts and outcomes to him, peace followed.

On February 21, 2008, we tried one more type of eye drop. If the eye did not respond to that, then it would have to come out. When I asked what would keep the eye from responding, I was reminded that when an eye dies, it either dies nicely like Cole's had, or it dies painfully. Any trauma to the eye, because it is full of scar tissue, could trigger the eye to go into the painful mode. Cole's eye was so full of scar tissue that the doctor could not see if there was inner eye damage from the branch. We would have to get that information from the pain Cole was experiencing. If these latest drops did not relieve the pain, then it would be obvious the branch did cause some inner eye damage and therefore must come out.

Praise God! He is good and faithful, as the drops began to work. The eye responded well and healed quickly after that. Cole now wears dark glasses all the time to protect his eyes. He has one pair for dress and one for play.

I finally felt like I could let out the big breath of air I had been holding in since January with all the sickness and accidents that caused the boys so much pain. No sooner did I breathe out than I had to breathe back in that same painful air when I noticed small drops of blood again in the bathroom. *Please, God, no more! I have complete trust and faith in you, but how much can one keep getting tested?* I thought of Job right away. I asked God to give me strength like Job. I knew Cole had this strength, the strength to make it through anything, but I was not sure if I did.

Cole's hypospadias had opened up again. This time, the surgery would have to be done in Minneapolis at the Minnesota Children's Hospital. Cole became very angry upon hearing this news. He snapped at everyone, frequently voicing his anger, and often just wanted to be left alone. Cole also prayed and talked to God, telling him how he was angry and frustrated with all that was his to deal with.

On a Wednesday night, Cole was at his youth group sharing his frustrations with his youth leader, who was ministering to and praying with Cole. At that exact same time, Mike was out of town on a job and was eating at a coworker's mom's house. As he ate, he noticed a plaque on the wall. The words that Mike read were, "God does not give us the things we can handle, God helps us handle the things we are given."

As Mike read those words, words he felt God had placed before him, he was also being ministered to. When Mike came home, he shared with Cole the words he had read. As they talked, they discovered that those words entered Mike's vision at the same time Cole was with his youth leader. They were thrilled to know that even when the family is apart, God has ways of comforting each one in the same moments of time.

Cole took the words his dad brought home to heart. He felt God was not going to leave him but instead was asking Cole to draw closer to him. He felt God's reassurances that he was with him and would be no matter what happened now or in the future. This helped Cole gain back his positive attitude. He was still angry and scared, but his trust in God was complete.

When it was time to take Cole to Minnesota for his surgery, it was Mike who took him. We would be apart once again during our child's operation, but this time our roles were reversed. I stayed home with Clay so he would not miss any school, and Mike would be with Cole during the rigors of pre-surgery, post surgery, and all that is in between. This was not what we were used to, and it added to the anxiety we all were feeling.

The surgery game plan was to either fix the urethra if it was a small repair or, if a larger repair was needed, a suprapubic catheter would be put in from the stomach. With this information in my brain, I was educated and prepared in knowledge but not prepared in my heart.

During the surgery, I depended on phone calls from Mike to keep me updated. The minutes felt like hours before the phone would ring. The first call came. Surgery started. The second call came and I was not prepared for it. Cole's urethra had so much damage that the doctor had to do an entirely different procedure than what we were told and had planned for.

The urethra had to be cut back, and a new urine hole had to be made. To do this, they took a large skin graft from Cole's mouth. They took the skin from one cheek, behind his lower lip and up the next cheek, and applied that skin to the penis. The result was 120 stitches in his mouth and eighty stitches on his penis.

I was able to hold it together until I got off the phone, but then the tears flowed freely. I was instantly filled with anger. Could not *one* surgery go simply? *How much loss and pain does Cole have to go through? Why does every part of him have to be different?*

After the surgery, Mike called me and said all went well and that they would be staying two nights in the hospital. The first night I talked to Cole, he was quiet because talking was very painful. When I talked to him about the surgery, he was quiet again, not because of the pain in his mouth but because of the hurt and frustration of loss. As the days went by and Cole was home again, he was able to talk about it more and with less emotion. It was so empowering watching Cole's faith through all of this. Sure he was going through every emotion possible from pain and fear to anger. Yet he never lost hope or trust in God. Clay also was blessed by Cole's strength; as he would say, "If Cole can do this, Mom, I can do anything also."

Mike had to show me how to take care of Cole since I was not there after the surgery. I have always been the stronger one. Blood, stitches, needles, tests…nothing could faze me any longer—until now.

I did my best to remain in control because I did not want to scare Cole, but what I saw made my stomach drop. The surgery left him covered in stitches, and blood was in his catheter. Mike showed me what all needed to be done, and I watched and listened carefully. When he was finished, I walked casually to the bathroom, where I threw up and began to cry. I did not tell anyone where I was or what I was doing. I did not want to worry Mike or scare Cole.

The nights were not easy. Cole had a small bag that would fill up with urine and needed to be changed every two hours and sometimes even every hour. Sleep quickly became a desperate need for both Cole and me. After a few nights of this, I called the doctor and was able to get a larger bag. This allowed us to get three to four hours of continual sleep at night.

Every day, Cole became stronger, and even though he was struggling with missing so many of his last days and events of the sixth grade, his spirits were high. The spring days were nice, and we spent much of them sitting outside as I read *The Chronicles of Narnia* to him.

I can do everything through him who gives me strength.

Philippians 4:13

I am the Lord, the God of all mankind. Is anything too hard for me?

Jeremiah 32:27

Graduation

Despite the days missed of school and the fact that he still had his catheter in, Cole was able to attend his sixth grade graduation. We walked into the gymnasium as a family. There were tables set up for the graduates and their families to sit at. We walked to one in the front of the room and sat down. I looked around at all Cole's friends who were dressed so nicely for this special event. Then I looked across the table at Cole. I was overwhelmed with a whirlwind of different emotions. He sat there, in his large pajama bottoms to accommodate his catheter, his mouth swollen, but still looking incredibly strong and very handsome.

A feeling of intense pride washed over me, mixing with concern and sadness that this wonderful event had to be overcast by the pain Cole was in. I knew that he had to be careful in all he did because of his catheter, and this added a tinge of aggravation to the event, but he was there. Despite missing the fun and activities of his last week of the sixth grade, he made it to the graduation itself. It was a perfect image of Cole's whole life, actually.

Cole has had to struggle through pain, surgeries, sickness, and fear throughout his years; but despite the many days, weeks, and months he had missed out on being your typical American boy, he did not miss out on life. He made it. He has done things I still cannot believe. Everything from walking, riding a scooter, knee boarding, skiing, four-wheeling, and going to camp; to fishing, bear hunting, and even mowing the lawn.

Joy settled into my heart as I went down memory lane, visiting the times when Cole was so little and I would hold him and rock him after some of his surgeries. During those intense moments, I never dreamed we would be at his sixth grade graduation, watching him as he walked to the front of the gym to receive the President's Award for Educational Achievement.

When I was told that Cole was blind, I remember thinking right away about marriage and proms and all the things that I thought he would not be able to do. I should have just trusted God in all that Cole *would* be able to do and just let God carry us on this journey. Back then, I could not see the future, and the unknown is always scary, especially when you live in a world that tells you things like, "It can't be done," or, "The statistics say ..."

That precious day I got the privilege to reminisce and see thirteen years' worth of what God can do. I have learned that it does not matter what the odds are or what medical experts tell us. God is in control. God knows what he is doing, even when we do not. Especially when we do not! I remember looking at Cole and realizing that he had learned this truth way before I had. I know I would not have been strong or brave enough to overcome all that he has. His faith and trust in God has pulled him through his many painful surgeries and tests. He may be blind, but he was able to see even before I could that with God all things are possible.

Remembering Cole, with diploma in hand, I got a glimpse of the man he is becoming. I saw a strong Christian husband and father. I know that despite setbacks and struggles God will lead him where he wants him to go, and I rest in the assurance that he will never leave Cole's side.

The memory of my gaze turns from Cole's amazing figure that was in front of me to Clay, sitting beside me. He too has had more than his share of trials. He too has overcome scary tests and painful surgery. Like his big brother, he has never been slowed down by these difficulties and continues to pursue his sports and other passions, succeeding in all he puts his mind to. I saw Clay sitting talking and supporting his brother, a role he has played all his life; however, he does it with pride and humility, as it must be hard sometimes living in the shadows of all Cole has been through.

I love how it felt having Mike seated next to me, and I am thankful for a partner so perfect for me. I rely on his strength and support as a husband, father, and best friend. I know his family is his first priority, and I find great security in this.

That day and every day since, I have felt that no woman has been blessed as much as me, surrounded by three wonderfully strong men with hearts for Christ, who desire to live their lives for him daily. I know that God has a special hold on us. No, we are not better than anyone else, but God has made his presence known to us by helping us through our very difficult journey. I may not know exactly why God has placed us on this particularly difficult path (and it is the *why* that torments all who must go through difficult times), but I do know that God has shown himself and what he can do through my family. As I really ponder on that, who am I to ever think that God owes me a why. I should just trust.

God has guided us through deep pain and great loss to immense joy and accomplishment. Friends with big hearts came in wonderful numbers. Times I never thought we would make it, we did. Things I thought would never happen did. All of it was answered prayers from those first nights of heartache given up to God from hospital floors.

So, as I think about us continuing on God's majestic journey, we will rest in God's love, we will welcome his strength, and we will continue to praise his name. For in all that we do not know, we do know that through him, truly, all things are possible. We just have to be willing to surrender it all before him!

"For I know the plans I have for you," declares the Lord, "plans to prosper you and not to harm you, plans to give you hope and a future. Then you will call upon me and come and pray to me, and I will listen to you. You will seek me and find me when you see me with all your heart. I will be found by you," declares the Lord, "and will bring you back from captivity."

Jeremiah 29:11–14

Epilogue

In life, most things come to an end. I am so excited to know that my family's life here on Earth is just the beginning of this great journey. I want to thank you for joining us on our travels thus far. I look forward to having you come along with us on the next great leg of this journey. Sometimes, as I look into the future and think where we should go on our next trip, all the worries of cost, location, weather, and timing come flooding into my mind. Sometimes this is so overwhelming that I do not even want to continue. The same occurs when I think of our medical journey; will Cole's cancer stay in remission? Will Cole get the miracle of sight? And will Clay's heart stay strong? When those thoughts start to inundate my every being, for a split second I just want to stop—stop thinking, stop moving, and stop planning—because it all seems too hard and painful to endure. Then I remember that God is in control. I do not need to plan; I need to surrender and trust him. He will be faithful in his own timing. So no matter what is involved in the travel plans and wherever our destination takes us, everything will be all right with him as our guide.

As I start this next journey, I can already see God's unending faithfulness. From Cole getting a long-time prayer and dream answered, to Clay experiencing great accomplishments, and Mike and I growing closer every day with the great joy of watching our boys become strong young men in Christ. I encourage you, my dear friend, to never stop looking forward to the next great journey lying before you, even if this destination is not what you hoped or dreamed for. May God bless your travels and make his presence known to you always.

Blessings in him.

"Walk by faith, not by sight" (2 Cor 5:7).

Talking with Cole

Do you remember any eye surgeries?

Yes, I remember sitting on Mom's lap and having to stick a needle through my eye. I remember Mom telling me to think of something peaceful. Even though this sounds very scary, I had no pain during this.

Do you remember the pain?

No, I don't remember the pain. I know I had it, but I do not remember it. I feel God saved me from all the pain.

How did it feel to know you had cancer?

At first it was scary. I thought, *Why is this happening to me?* Then I realized it was what it was. Maybe I just got used to it. I remember asking God, "Why me? What have I done to deserve this?"

What did it feel like to be on chemo?

Bad. It was like I could never remember anything; I was so out of it. I got so sick with headaches, sore throat, body aches, and nausea. I never was angry with God, but I can say I was frustrated with him and the situation.

What was it like going back to Otter Tail Lake?

At first I was nervous that I would get cancer again. Deep down, I was worried I was going to get sick again. But after we left, I knew it was time to move on with my life. I realized that I need to move on and trust God.

How has all of this affected your relationship with God?

It has taught me to trust God more and believe in him, that he is with me even when I am so sick. I trust him completely and could not make it without him. I am a stronger Christian because of everything I have been through. It just shows that he has a plan for everyone, even though we do not understand what is going on and cannot see the reasoning behind it all.

What were the angels like that you saw by the car after losing your eye?

There was a warming blue light that surrounded them, and they wore white robes. They did not speak. I was afraid of them at first, but once I realized who and what they were, I felt at ease. I think it was God's way of letting me know he is with me.

When was the first time you went to heaven? What was it like?

I don't remember the first time. I was only four. I remember seeing Steve and just had a feeling of who he was.

What was it like when you saw Bobby in heaven?

There was a lot of holy light and a big room (banquet hall) with lots of people. The people didn't have a human form, just beings of light. I could not hear much. Bobby never spoke out loud; it was like I just felt what he was saying.

Do you still go to heaven?

I went a few times after Bobby. I don't remember much except that there was a lot of light. I have not gone in a long time.

Do you wish to go again?

Some days I wish I could go. Sometimes I tell God I would like to go again, but I don't know if I can anymore.

Did you ever just want to die? Are you afraid of dying?

I tell God, "If you want me to go, I'll go. If you want me to stay, I'll stay. I am in your hands." When the pain was really bad, I wanted God to end it, even if that meant to die. I am not really afraid to die because I know it will be my time.

What do you want people to know about being blind?

It is like having your eyes closed all the time. At first it is scary, but then it gets better. When people first started asking me why I was blind, I would be sad or offended. But now I can talk about it. I am just like everyone else, I just cannot see, so I would like to be treated just like everyone else.

What do you want people to know about you?

If you go through things, let God guide you. I know that I have become a better person because of it all. Even though I am blind, I want to try different things and be a part of others' lives. I am a trustworthy person who just wants to serve God and bring others closer to him. I would like it if people would give me a chance and get to know me. People with disabilities are just like everyone else.

Talking with Clay

What do you remember about your heart surgery?
I remember just being very scared, and then after it was done, trusting God that he would always protect me.

Before the doctor found out about your heart, did you ever feel like something was wrong?
Yes, I always had this feeling when I would eat something and it would get stuck that something was wrong. I just felt it in my inner heart.

Do you remember the pain of heart surgery?
Yes, it hurt really bad to walk or move. I remember crying a lot. When I was on the breathing machine, it was so scary because I did not know I would wake up on one, and I could not talk, so I thought, *What did they do to me?*
Then they told me they were going to take it (the breathing tube) out, and I was so scared because I could not ask them if it would hurt. I was so happy because I thought the tube would hurt, but it did not hurt to be taken out.

Are you afraid of something being wrong with your heart now?
Not anymore.

How did you feel when Cole got cancer?

I felt very sad, and I was afraid he was going to die. I was angry with God and wanted him to take the cancer away. I started not to trust him.

Did watching Cole make going through your heart surgery harder or easier?

It gave me peace because I thought, *If he can do this, so can I.* Plus, he gave me great tips.

Is it hard to be in Cole's shadow in the sense that he gets so much more attention sometimes?

No, because I feel like I am the lucky one, not being blind, and I would not want to have to go through what he did just to get attention off of him and on to me.

How has God been a part of your life?

I just know he is a big part of my life. I trust him now.

What do you want people to know about you?

I really do not want people to know I had heart surgery. Instead, I want them to know that I am an honest, Christian guy that will help them and be kind to them.

Talking with Mike

How did you feel when you found out about Cole's disability?

I felt very lonely and lost. I did not know where or who to turn to. I also was very mad, although I did not know who to be mad at.

How did you feel when Cole and Laura were in Arizona so much during the first few months of Cole's life?

I felt very lonely and detached from my wife and son. For a while, I felt like I did not even have a family. I also felt very helpless so far away from them.

How did you feel when they first found cancer on Cole's kidney?

I felt that Cole had been through enough and wondered how much more he could take and would have to take. I also wondered if this would be his time to pass on.

How did you feel after the miracle of the healing?

When the doctor told us it was gone, I felt numb because I was ready for the worst news possible.

Once Cole lost his sight, did you ever feel scared or frustrated?

I felt all of the above and more. Through Cole's life, it has been one thing after another and so ongoing.

How did you deal with it?

I did not know what I, as his dad, was supposed to do. So I have taken things day by day and learn more with every step I take.

Did you feel close to Laura, or did this cause a gap between you?

I felt for a long time we grew apart because we put so much time and emotion into this journey. I do know that I could have never made it through this without her.

What were your emotions during the first few weeks of Cole having cancer the second time?

Very angry at everything and everyone.

How did his chemo affect you?

I felt helpless once again as a parent, watching my child wilt away and become very fragile.

Did you pray a lot?

For a while, I did; but as things went on, I drew apart from God and was wondering why he could let all of this happen to such a good boy.

What were your inner thoughts when they told you Clay would need surgery?

I was mad and scared because I did not know if he would be okay. I was scared, but at the same time, this all did not seem real to me. This was not supposed to happen to Clay; I thought of him as healthy.

Did your faith grow or fall away during Clay's heart surgery?

My faith fell even farther away when this happened.

What do you want people to know about you?

That I am a father and husband, just like others. I would do anything for my family, and I love them very much.

Prayer of Salvation

The Bible says that if you confess with your mouth Jesus is Lord and believe in your heart that God raised him from the dead, you will be saved (Romans 10:9 NIV).

For "Everyone who calls on the name of the Lord will be saved" (Romans 10:13 NIV).

God's greatest gift to us is eternal salvation, through the death of his Son, Jesus Christ. Through this salvation, we receive many benefits and blessings from God, the greatest being eternal life with God. God makes this available to all who believe and confess Jesus as their Lord and Savior. Does being saved mean you are perfect? No; however, you are forgiven, and you will want to strive to be more like Christ every day. So if you are ready to have a personal relationship with Christ and receive this great gift, please pray the prayer below.

> Lord Jesus, I believe you are the son of God. Thank you for dying on the cross for my sins. Please forgive all my sins and give me the gift of eternal life. I ask you into my life and heart to be my personal Lord and Savior, and I want to serve you always. In Jesus' precious name. Amen.

listen|imagine|view|experience

AUDIO BOOK DOWNLOAD INCLUDED WITH THIS BOOK!

In your hands you hold a complete digital entertainment package. Besides purchasing the paper version of this book, this book includes a free download of the audio version of this book. Simply use the code listed below when visiting our website. Once downloaded to your computer, you can listen to the book through your computer's speakers, burn it to an audio CD or save the file to your portable music device (such as Apple's popular iPod) and listen on the go!

How to get your free audio book digital download:

1. Visit www.tatepublishing.com and click on the e|LIVE logo on the home page.
2. Enter the following coupon code:
   25fa-07cf-7cdc-bac5-df8d-9b1c-03b4-638c
3. Download the audio book from your e|LIVE digital locker and begin enjoying your new digital entertainment package today!